Suicide (

The Story

Joy Hibbins

ISBN: 978-1-326-39604-6

Suicide Crisis is a company and a charity

www.suicidecrisis.co.uk

The money raised from the sale of this book will go directly to Suicide Crisis, to help people who are at risk of suicide.
Cover photograph by kind permission of the Gloucestershire Echo.

This is the story of how a mental health patient set up the first Suicide Crisis Centre of its kind in Britain, providing face to face intensive and ongoing care to people at risk of suicide. The charity has never had a suicide of a client under its care. We have been providing services for over two years.

I think it probably took a person with mental health issues, who had recently been in suicidal crisis, to set this up. I knew how much the creation of a Suicide Crisis Centre mattered, and I would fight to set it up with a determination to overcome each barrier that was put in our way – against a backdrop of scepticism and incredulity, displayed by people in positions of power and influence, that a person like me was even thinking of doing this.

Prior to 2012 I had no mental health diagnoses – now I have several. Those who assumed that my mental health issues made me less able failed to recognise that, in some ways, the opposite is true.

The sceptics failed to realise that it was my experience of being suicidal that informs my work now. Those of us who have been at the point of suicide, or who have attempted suicide, carry a knowledge and an understanding of what it is like to be in that place that many clinicians will never have. I believe that my mental health issues give me an additional dimension that I didn't have before. I do not believe that the person that I was before 2012 (a person without mental health diagnoses or suicidal history) would have been able to set up this charity or run it.

I don't want to minimise the effects of mental illness, though. All three of my mental health conditions carry an increased risk of suicide. In the period that our charity has been offering services, there have been times when I have been at risk myself, and needed to take time out. Despite working tenaciously to try to help our clients stay alive, I found it much harder to keep myself alive, at times. I did not know that I had bipolar. I was only diagnosed in February 2015. All I knew was that there were times when I would fall into such a deep depression, that I was a risk to myself. I wish that I had been diagnosed earlier.

I need to take you back to 2012 to explain how this all started.

There are some people who say that they cannot understand or imagine what is like to be suicidal. However, I think it is perhaps that they have not encountered the unique set of circumstances that might push them into suicidal crisis. A single catastrophic and unimaginable event may destabilise you and propel you into crisis. Suicidality usually involves a complex interplay of different factors, and additional circumstances that occur around the time of the catastrophic event may make us more vulnerable to suicidal thoughts. Similarly, depression can affect any one of us. During a depressive illness, you may experience such intense emotional pain that life may seem unbearable. Depression can alter your thoughts and perceptions in such a way that you may no longer believe that you have any value, or that your continued existence matters. You are no longer thinking as you usually would, because the illness has temporarily changed the way that you view yourself, the people you love and the world in general. I don't feel that any of us is immune from experiencing suicidal crisis at some point in our lives, no matter how much we may believe, in our current circumstances, that it could never happen to us.

Before 2012 I had never attempted suicide. I have now attempted suicide several times, in ways that I could never have imagined doing.

I had also had no contact with mental health services prior to 2012. I now have a detailed knowledge of community mental health care, crisis care and inpatient care in a psychiatric hospital, from personal experience. I firmly believe that my personal experiences of the different psychiatric services, from a patient's perspective, and my experiences of being admitted to hospital after suicide attempts, give me a depth of knowledge of services that most people who work with suicidal clients don't have.

The traumatic experience which changed my life came ten days after my mother died. I had become her full time carer for the last two years of her life because she became increasingly unwell with Parkinson's Disease. Her life was happy until her last three weeks. She always wanted to live – right to the end. Despite needing help with every aspect of her life from washing to eating to walking, her quality of life was good. She was loved and cared for. And she was an optimist – always. I used to be, too.

I retain some of my former optimism. Although I find it difficult to be optimistic about my own life, because I feel so profoundly changed by the events of the past three years, I retain my optimism for our clients' futures and for their survival. I always believe that they can survive, and that they will go on to contribute in a positive way in the world, affecting people's lives for the better. We see how unique they are. Our clients are some of the most caring, sensitive and helpful people that you could meet. They give me so much hope for the future.

My life is now divided into two parts: the period before 28th March 2012, and the period after 28th March 2012. A single event fractured my life. I am profoundly changed by it and my life has been profoundly changed by it.

During the event itself, it was as if my mind separated. There was a part of my mind that was experiencing shock, terror, fear, horror, incomprehension and unbearable emotional distress. But there was a part of my mind – a smaller part – that had separated out and was remaining rational and focused. I was trying to hold onto the smallest detail of the person's face, to focus on any aspect that might help me afterwards, or help me understand what had happened. I can even remember telling myself "You must remember this detail, because it may help you to make sense of what has happened."

In retrospect, I think this was my first experience of dissociation, which psychiatrists diagnosed later. Clinicians frequently commented, in the months after the trauma, that there was a "disconnect between my thoughts and my emotions", at times. The way that I responded, during the traumatic event itself, appears to show this same disconnect. During one of the most shocking events of my life, a part of my brain was commenting quite rationally and unemotionally, focusing on taking in the finest details, in an attempt to block out the deeply painful emotions that I was experiencing and help myself make sense of what I had experienced.

Even during the traumatic event itself, I was aware that my life would never be the same. I knew that nothing would ever be the same again. My mind processed so much, in such a short space of time.

There was a sense of being trapped, being captive, and that can often make the subsequent post-traumatic reaction worse.

I developed symptoms of Post-Traumatic Stress Disorder almost immediately, although I did not recognise them as such. I was reliving the trauma, day and night. Images of the event would appear in my head, in my dreams. I couldn't escape from it and realised that I would never be able to escape from it.

On around the third day after the event, I started to develop an inexplicable fear. At first, I could not clarify what it was that I was afraid of. It started in my home, one evening. It was a sense of terror. I couldn't sit with my back to a door. I was afraid of something or someone – but couldn't pin down what or who. As the hours went by, it became clear that the source of my fear was upstairs. It was a fear that there were dark forces (malevolent forces) upstairs. This continued for several days.

I did not seek medical help during this time. I had no idea what was happening to me. Psychiatrists subsequently felt that the belief that there may be dark forces upstairs constituted a psychotic episode.

I had never had a psychotic episode in my life before. Initially, when a psychiatrist gave me his view that this had been a psychotic episode, I was hugely in denial. Surely this couldn't have happened. I now recognise and accept it. I think that it shows the impact of the traumatic event.

Most of us fear psychosis so much. It is perhaps what we fear most, in terms of mental illness. Now that I have experienced it, it is not psychosis itself that I fear, but rather the fear that I could have another psychotic episode which might, this time, lead to my being detained for a prolonged period under the Mental Health Act (sectioned). If I had sought help, in the days after the traumatic event, it is likely that I would have been sectioned. I have had experience, in the past three years, of being detained for short periods, not knowing how long it would be before I would be released. I know the sense of total powerlessness that you feel, at that time. My fear is that, one day, I might be sectioned for a period of weeks or months. It is the consequences of having another psychotic episode that I fear.

In the first few days after the event, I wanted to die, but my thoughts were focused on the possibility of having an accident that would lead to my death. I used to cycle everywhere. People have accidents on bikes all the time. I desperately wished that a careless driver would be the cause of an accident that would end my life.

One day I was cycling towards a roundabout, and could see a lorry driving at high speed towards it, at the next junction. He was driving far too fast. I had right of way on the roundabout. As I cycled past the junction that the speeding lorry was approaching, I suddenly slowed, giving him every opportunity, if he continued at the same speed, to hit me. He braked suddenly. I had not planned this action, before I saw the speeding lorry, but it was a decision in the moment. It felt as if the opportunity to die that I so desperately craved was being presented to me in the form of the speeding lorry.

From that point onwards, the desire to die increased. I felt that I could not live with the knowledge of what I had experienced on the 28th March. Thoughts of suicide repeatedly entered my head.

The first descent into crisis happened very quickly, a few days later. In the hours leading up to the crisis, I had thoughts of suicide, but no focused intent to harm myself. Within the space of an hour, I changed from having no immediate intent, to having my suicide method in my hand, and the intention of using it to end my life. It had not been planned at all. I stood for a few moments, holding it, ready to act. Then I recall grasping the edge of the kitchen sink, trying to steady myself. I am not sure how long I remained there, but I eventually called the out of hours doctor.

These impulsive acts are particularly dangerous. I have subsequently experienced the absolute tunnel vision of focused suicidal intent, which can come on very quickly, usually as a result of a triggering incident. There is nothing else but that focused intent. Everything else has disappeared. The people who you love are no longer in your consciousness. You are no longer able to consider them, or consider the impact of your suicide upon them. All the aspects of your life that would usually prevent you from ending your life are blocked out.

I was asked to come to the out of hours GP surgery at the hospital immediately. The GP spoke to me for an hour, and arranged my first contact with the NHS crisis team, who support people at risk of suicide.

Crisis team members are usually psychiatric nurses, although the team may include social workers who have experience of working in mental health. They work in the community and either one or two members of the team provide home visits to patients under their care, who are in mental health crisis. Initially these may be daily visits, usually for an hour, and the visits become less frequent as the patient's situation improves. In some cases, there may be more than one visit a day.

Crisis teams were created as an alternative to admission to psychiatric hospital.

There was no one from the crisis team available to come out to assess me until the next day, so they phoned to determine whether I would be safe in the hours before their visit.

The following day two members of the team came out to see me, assessed me, and felt that I did not meet the criteria to be taken onto their caseload. However, they gave me the crisis team phone numbers and advised me to call them if I felt at risk again.

They had not been unduly concerned about the "dark forces" that I had sensed a few days earlier, and did not appear to equate them with psychotic perceptions. It was several weeks before a psychiatrist identified them, in retrospect, as psychotic.

It was a week later that I called them again, on a Saturday evening. They felt that my situation had deteriorated, and came out to assess me the same evening. They explored what I had done in the days since I last saw them. I acknowledged that I had been to see a solicitor to make a will. It had been drawn up and I needed to return to the solicitor's office on Monday, in order to sign it. I had carried out other final acts. At one point, they focused on the calendar on the kitchen wall. They commented that, in the weeks leading up to the approaching Monday, the calendar was full of events and reminders. After Monday, the calendar was empty, they remarked. I was not conscious of this at all, and was astonished that they had noticed it.

At that point I was assessed as being at high risk of suicide, and was taken onto their caseload.

In the days that followed one of the psychiatric nurses who undertook the assessment that weekend came to see me. He had empathy, treated me with respect, and appeared genuinely concerned. He revealed that he had also lost a parent and, although it was the recent trauma that was triggering my suicidal intent, he was aware that grief must be contributing to my emotional turmoil. My impression was that he had been profoundly affected by the death of his parent, and identified with that aspect of my current situation.

I soon discovered that it was highly unusual to see the same crisis team nurse on consecutive days. I never experienced that kind of continuity of care again, or that empathic understanding, under the crisis team. By the end of the week I was seeing different nurses every day, a pattern which continued throughout the remainder of my time with them. They appeared detached and distant in their approach. On one occasion, a crisis team member gave a very pointed representation of this clinical distance by arriving at my home, entering the dining room and pulling a chair away from the table, where I sat, to the very far end of the room. He sat right against the wall, at the furthest distance possible from me. It was unsettling, disconcerting, and I struggled to speak to him at all.

When a crisis team member arrived at my home, it was often the case that they had only read the notes of the preceding visit, and had no real knowledge of my situation or why I was suicidal. This meant that I was often expected to explain, again and again to different nurses, why I was suicidal.

If you have experienced trauma, it is not helpful to have to repeat detail of the traumatic event over and over again, to different people. It is also virtually impossible to build trust with members of their team, if you are repeatedly seeing different nurses.

It is often the case, if you have experienced a deeply traumatic event, that you experience a profound loss of trust in people, and a lack of trust in the world in general. It can be hugely challenging to build trust with one person, so the prospect of a large team can seem overwhelming.

A person will generally be under the care of the crisis team for around two to four weeks, although it is more likely to be closer to two weeks. I remained on their caseload for several weeks, as the crisis team psychiatrist was reluctant to discharge me. He described himself as being "professionally puzzled" by my case. One of my friends, who works in psychiatric services in another part of the country, remarked, somewhat cynically, that this was translated as: "We don't know what's wrong with you."

It was in May 2012 that a member of the crisis team first noticed that I may be experiencing dissociation. It was a social worker who was part of the crisis team.

The second weekend in May had been particularly difficult for me and I had awoken on that sunny Sunday morning and made a decision to kill myself. There were things that I needed to put in order, including arranging a headstone for my mother's grave, and so I made a decision that I would kill myself the following Saturday, the 19th May. The number nineteen appealed to me, since my nineteenth year had been one of the happiest of my life. At the age of nineteen I worked in southern France for a few months and then started university in the same year, a blissfully happy and exciting time for me.

The day that I made my decision, the 13th May, was extraordinary, in terms of the sense of elation that I felt. I felt absolutely euphoric. It was an intensely bright, sunny day and I was, for the first time since March, able to enjoy a day, since I knew that I would soon be released from the pain that I experienced, and that my life would end within days.

Early in the week I went to order a headstone for my mother's grave. I chose a pale grey headstone and asked for them to create the inscription in white lettering, because my mother had loved white flowers. There was an abundance of white roses in her garden.

They advised me that the arrangement for payment for a headstone was an initial payment at the time of ordering it, with the full balance required a few weeks later, when the headstone was completed, so that the customer could check that the firm had carried out the inscription correctly.

This was out of the question, and I insisted on paying the full balance at the time of ordering it.

I was still under the crisis team. In the middle of that week I disclosed my plan to one of them. I spoke about the euphoria that I had experienced at the weekend, when I made my decision. I described my absolute intent to end my life, but, at the same time, expressed my surprise that I was proceeding in an apparently detached, quite calculating way to plan to die on the 19th: "It's so cold and planned. This seems so out of character because I'm usually a more emotional person." It was that element of detachment – being able to almost stand outside myself and, despite my very focused intention to die, being able to comment as an outsider on what I was feeling and doing, and how out of character it was – that led the crisis team to bring out a psychiatrist.

A crisis team member told the psychiatrist that they had called him out because I seemed to be a "witness to my emotions". She and the psychiatrist spent an hour with me, at the end of which the psychiatrist expressed his concerns that there was a "disconnect" between my thoughts and emotions.

Later that day I called the crisis team and asked them what he meant by this. They agreed to leave a message for the psychiatrist to call me. When he returned my call, he explained that "it had the feel of dissociation".

This was confirmed by other psychiatrists over time.

Dissociation is an extraordinary mechanism that the brain employs, in order to protect you from emotions that may be too painful to bear.

The focus of the crisis team turned to the issue of the date of my planned suicide, since I had not revealed that. I felt that it might be taken from me, if I revealed it. I felt that they might prevent me from doing it. A part of me wanted to tell them, since I felt under increasing pressure from them to do so, but another part of me wanted to protect my opportunity to die.

In the early hours of the 18th I called the crisis team. By chance, the psychiatric nurse, with whom I had engaged in my first few days under their care, was the one who answered.

In my psychiatric records, he describes me as being in a "mixed affective state, superficially emotional but presenting as calm and controlled underneath the initial presentation". I recall it as a strange conversation. We moved tentatively towards the subject of the day of my planned suicide, and I eventually revealed that it was the following day.

Suddenly it was as if everything moved into high gear. Psychiatric hospital admission was mentioned and I became very fearful. I instantly regretted revealing the date to him.

My fear of admission to psychiatric hospital meant that the crisis team agreed to support me at home on my planned suicide date.

On the morning of my planned suicide, I had an extremely unsettling experience. It was as if I felt the presence of death, right beside me, in the form of a physical barrier that I was being invited to cross.

A psychiatric nurse came out and made clear his view that I should be admitted to psychiatric hospital over the weekend, for safety. I refused, though. He gave me sedating medication and put in place a safety plan for the weekend, which involved additional visits to my home and phone calls.

The 'presence of death' experience is particularly memorable, but I had many other strange and inexplicable experiences during the spring and summer of 2012. Many of them seemed to be dissociative episodes, where the world around me appeared altered.

Sometimes it was I who appeared altered. On one occasion I was at a garden centre, looking for plants to adorn the garden, and I suddenly had the sensation of being much taller, around eight feet tall, I would estimate. I could feel that I was much higher above the ground. On another occasion, I was walking across a bridge and realised that I no longer felt that I was in contact with the bridge. It was as if I was hovering somewhere above it. It became incredibly difficult to make my way across it, and I had to focus on placing each foot very firmly on the ground, moving very slowly, concentrating on feeling the sensation of my foot pressing into the bridge, and watching my feet so that I could see that I was making contact.

I have also had the experience of feeling as if I am outside my own body, as if I am standing to the right of me, and I find this one of the most unnerving dissociative experiences.

It is extraordinary that the brain is able to make these sensations and perceptions feel totally real. It is not a loss of reality, as in psychosis, but an altered reality, since you are aware that the dissociative experiences are not reality.

In those early days, I felt like a visitor in mental health land. There was an element of fascination at being in a world that was unknown to me, where extraordinary things happened, particularly in terms of dissociation. It was like being taken on a journey that I was not controlling. I was being taken along as a passenger on a train. I was not driving it and had no idea where I was going to be taken next. That was frightening at times, but hugely exciting, too. I never knew what would happen next or what I would experience.

I now live in mental health land. I am no longer a visitor.

I still regularly experience a disconnect between my thoughts and emotions, and it is this manifestation of dissociation that has always been the most prevalent, in my case.

This 'disconnect' has sometimes protected me from emotional distress in my work at our Suicide Crisis Centre. There are times when a client may speak about something that may be quite triggering to me, since it can reconnect me with my own trauma, but I am protected by my dissociative response of disconnecting from my emotions.

GPs felt that I was showing symptoms of Post-Traumatic Stress Disorder in the summer of 2012, but the crisis team did not pursue this, when I raised the possibility with them. I was not assessed for the condition until July 2013, over a year after the trauma, and this assessment only occurred after intervention from a friend, who is a clinician in another part of the country. She had been carrying out assessments for PTSD for many years, and it was a particular area of interest for her. She carried out the Impact of Events Scale Assessment on me, which is a widely-used diagnostic tool for PTSD, and my score was 75, which indicated severe post-traumatic symptoms. This led to an assessment within my local mental health trust, and a diagnosis of PTSD by a psychiatrist.

Unfortunately it was not an enduring diagnosis, and a psychiatrist disagreed with the assessment result a few months later. It was only in May 2015 that the diagnosis was reinstated, when a very senior Oxford psychiatrist reported his view that I was experiencing a post-traumatic syndrome. This was added to my bipolar diagnosis from February 2015.

It is only in this year, three years after the traumatic event, that my mental health issues have been understood. The failure to diagnose and treat, in the months (and indeed years) after the trauma, has been catastrophic. It meant that I repeatedly experienced episodes of bipolar depression, which were not recognised as such, and in which I became a suicide risk. It meant that I did not receive treatment according to NICE guidelines, for mental conditions which carried an increased risk of suicide. In particular, I did not receive trauma-focused therapy.

My dissociative experiences appeared to be worsening towards the end of the summer of 2012. I had a sense of disconnection from the person that I used to be, before 2012, as if that person no longer existed. I felt that only the outer shell of her remained. I felt that I only continued to exist as a physical form.

My PTSD symptoms remained severe, and, as I was undiagnosed, I received no support in managing the symptoms. It felt a torturous existence, and my suicidal intent increased.

At the time of my first suicide attempt, in October 2012, I had done little research into different methods. There had been a well-publicised suicide in the media of a high-profile individual, and I was aware of the method that he had used, so it was in my consciousness. It appealed to me, because it appeared to be a method which allowed a greater degree of control over my death than other methods. I understood the processes that would occur in the body, with this method, and how they would lead to my death.

I had ruled out medication overdose because I did not understand the processes that would occur in the body after taking it. I would have no control over those processes, once the medication was inside me. I had the sense that the chemicals would overwhelm my body, acting in ways that I could not predict or imagine, creating internal chaos and perhaps unimaginable pain.

In the hours leading up to my first suicide attempt, I experienced a greater fear than I had expected. I had no fear of death, but, in order to reach that destination, I had to overcome the barrier which protects us from harming ourselves. Our natural instinct is not to harm ourselves. I remember talking to myself quietly, reassuring myself, in the moments leading up to the attempt.

It was difficult, it was painful and it did far less damage than I had expected. My subsequent research revealed that it is extremely unreliable, and there are very few documented cases of suicide with this method.

It was distressing not to have achieved the outcome that I intended, and I called a self-harm helpline. Although these calls are anonymous, the service provider can arrange for the call to be traced, if they have concerns about the safety of the caller. The call handler was concerned that I had been injured and, having been unable to accurately determine the extent of my injury, she had the call traced and requested a police welfare check.

Two police officers visited me at home and took me to the general hospital for treatment of my injury and psychiatric assessment. There are psychiatric liaison teams based within general hospitals.

My experience of the psychiatric liaison team in the general hospital has been positive. I have found the psychiatric nurses who work within that team empathic, caring, and focused on trying to ensure that the patient has the right mental health support on leaving the hospital. Our clients report having had similar positive experiences.

The police officers ensured that I was checked into A&E and then announced their intention to leave. However, the officers warned me that, if I left the hospital and they were called out again to search for me as a missing person, they would take me to psychiatric hospital. I later learned that a patient should never be threatened with psychiatric hospital in this way. It should not be used as a threat, or a penalty, if you fail to abide by what a police officer wants you to do.

The experience of waiting to be assessed in A&E, when you are feeling suicidal, can be extremely stressful, and people frequently leave. You may be in a crowded waiting room, surrounded by people, and find it overwhelming. Or you may be placed in a totally different environment, and left alone in a room, sometimes for hours, and the feeling of solitude in a stark, clinical environment can be too much to bear.

Although the hospital staff wanted to admit me to a ward overnight, to ensure my safety, there were no beds available and I was told that I would be kept in A&E overnight. I felt that I could not remain in that environment any longer since it was adding to my distress, and I left.

As I walked up the road, I recalled the police officer's threat of psychiatric hospital. However, I received a text message from Gloucestershire Police which reassured me. The text read: "GlosPolice. Please ring 101 quoting incident 33. We have concerns for your welfare and just want to know you're okay. Thanks Joy." I walked home and shortly afterwards the two police officers arrived at my house. One of the officers told me immediately that they were taking me to the psychiatric hospital. They asked me no questions to assess my mental state or my mental capacity.

I had never been to a psychiatric hospital and I was shocked and afraid. I started to back away from him and retreated to the far end of the kitchen, and he took hold of me, at the top of my arms, pressing his hands into me. He told me that they would be taking me there. I begged them to take me back to the general hospital instead. I was not angry or violent or abusive. I was submissive. I fell to the ground as he was holding me, which was clearly a submissive act, and he forced me back up to my feet. The officer held me by my arms as they took me to the police van, and I was placed in a cage in the back of the van. I said nothing while I was in there. I was seated on a bench with no safety belt and just remained very still. The police officers did not communicate with me in any way. It appeared to be a cage of reinforced glass. It was extremely frightening being in a reinforced cage, with no communication or reassurance from the officers.

Several weeks later I asked a police officer how people usually behave, when they are placed in a cage in the back of a police van. He told me that they usually kick or punch the sides of the cage, are abusive, angry and violent. I sat totally silently, wishing that I had the means to kill myself in the van. I should never have been placed in a cage. I was a vulnerable person who was unwell.

The events of that night became the subject of a legal case which the police settled before it went to court. On the advice of my solicitors, I sued Gloucestershire Constabulary for assault and battery, false imprisonment, misfeasance in public office and negligence. Eighty per cent of the settlement money went to our charity, Suicide Crisis. That was the reason why I pursued the case. I intended that the money would benefit our charity, which needed funds so much.

The police officers took me to the 136 suite at the psychiatric hospital. The psychiatric staff asked me where I was when the police had detained me, and I explained that I had been in my kitchen. They immediately told me that I should not have been brought to a 136 suite since it appeared that I had been wrongly detained. You cannot be detained under a section 136 in your own home. It is a section that should be used when a person is in a public place, and there are concerns that the person may have a mental disorder and needs to be taken to a place of safety. However, the psychiatric staff told me that they still had to proceed with the assessment, now that I had been brought there.

The 136 suite is a small, enclosed, secure unit at the side of the psychiatric hospital. The heavy exterior doors are locked and there is no possibility of escape. I felt trapped, imprisoned. I was informed that I would be assessed under the Mental Health Act and I knew that this could lead to my being detained for a longer period within the psychiatric hospital, possibly for months.

The only occasion that I have self-harmed as a release for emotions that became unbearable (rather than as a suicide attempt) is when I was in the 136 suite.

I had been left alone in a room while the psychiatric nurses sat in the office, waiting for the assessing psychiatrists and the AMHP (Approved Mental Health Practitioner) to arrive. My bag had not been removed, and I found an object within it that I could use to harm myself.

When a psychiatric nurse came into the room and saw that I had harmed myself, her focus was upon the drops of blood that were falling onto the floor, and the mess that was being created, as a result. She immediately chastised me for "dripping blood onto the floor." She showed no concern for me, my injury or my mental state at the time, which had led me to self-harm.

Eventually the psychiatrists and AMHP arrived. I was assessed under the Mental Health Act, found not to be detainable, and was released. One of the psychiatrists told me that he would be referring me to a psychiatrist for further assessment as an outpatient, because he was puzzled by my presentation. This was now becoming a recurring theme.

Although I initially respected the psychiatrists' honesty in expressing their "puzzlement", I was becoming increasingly concerned that no one would be able to understand me or provide relevant treatment or help.

I was told that I would be assessed by a psychiatrist who was highly respected, very experienced and who had a particular interest in dissociation, which had been the only part of my presentation that the psychiatrists had agreed upon, so far. He would also consider whether psychological therapy would be appropriate.

I attended the appointment and he asked me to come in and sit down. He sat directly opposite me during the assessment. I felt that I was under intense scrutiny, as if in a laboratory. He commented on my physical reactions during the assessment, in particular that I would "shiver" at times. I tried to explain that they were shudders and that I was recoiling from the images that were entering my mind as flashbacks.

The notes that he made, which are in my psychiatric records, show that my sense of disconnection from my past self was such that I no longer felt that I was a person. I knew that I existed, but I seemed to exist as an automaton, and my sense of having a personality had gone.

He questioned me about the "dark forces" that I had sensed in the days after the traumatic incident and asked if I was religious. I explained that I had no strong religious conviction, had no idea if there was a God, but that I respected the different religions and had found it interesting in my previous life to learn about different religions from my adult students. I had been a teacher of English as a Second Language. It had been fascinating to learn from them about Buddhism and Hinduism. I spoke about the festival of light, in particular. The psychiatrist wrote in his notes: "Is she lost in darkness?"

He said that he thought that psychological therapy might be helpful at some time in the future but he didn't seem to think that it was currently indicated. His verbal summary at the end didn't include PTSD, despite the fact that I was experiencing flashbacks during the appointment. I was devastated because the post-traumatic symptoms were so overwhelming. I didn't tell him how distressed I felt by his conclusions, and left quietly.

If I was lost in darkness, it felt as if they were going to leave me there.

I felt an increasing sense of despair and, in the days that followed, I took two overdoses. The second was described by a psychiatrist as a very substantial overdose. This was a method that I had ruled out previously. However, a person who is highly distressed, and intent on suicide, will use methods that they would not previously have contemplated using. The very fact that a person may use a method, that has previously been abhorrent to them, suggests that they are in a very different place, mentally, from usual.

Neither of these attempts was planned. In the early part of the day I had no intention of taking them and both appeared to happen very suddenly. I must have made a decision within minutes, and then taken them. They appear, in retrospect, to have been impulsive attempts. I have no recollection of the thoughts or emotions that I was experiencing in the moments leading up to either attempt. It's unsettling to have no recollection of this as I recall clearly the emotions that I felt leading up to my first attempt a month earlier, which I had been planning from early that day.

Impulsive attempts are extremely dangerous. With a planned attempt, there may be time for you to change your mind, and time for thoughts to enter your mind of the consequences of your death and the people who will be affected. This can prevent an attempt. However, even in a planned suicide, a person may be so mentally unwell that they are unable to see the consequences or the effect of their death upon other people. If you are clinically depressed, your thought processes and your view of the world may be entirely altered. Our clients frequently describe feeling that it would be better for the people around them, including those who love them, if they were dead. They feel that they are a "burden" to everyone and often describe their belief that people will quickly get over their death. Their illness can prevent them from seeing that those who love them would be devastated by their death, and would be profoundly affected by it for the rest of their life.

Although I have no recollection of events in the twenty four hours after the second overdose, I now know what happened. A nurse from my GP surgery, who always visited me on a Thursday, came on a Wednesday that week and found me. I was not expecting her and had not been advised that she would be visiting on a different day. Afterwards she explained that she had been informed by my GP about the previous overdose and that is why she visited a day earlier.

According to the nurse, I took a long time to answer the door, and was very unsteady on my feet. I was giggling a lot and, embarrassingly and inappropriately, I was saying "It's like being drunk." I am mortified by that now, because I had made an attempt on my life. Nothing could be more serious than that. She called for an ambulance and tried to keep me conscious. I was conscious when the ambulance arrived.

The drugs that I took wiped my memory of the next twenty four hours. I have vague recollections of the following evening when I was still in the hospital bed, talking to the crisis team. Apparently I told them that I was going to leave the hospital and take another overdose. I have no recollection of saying that but I accept that it is totally possible that I did. That stated intention led to my being assessed under the Mental Health Act by two psychiatrists and an Approved Mental Health Practitioner (a social worker).

I remember very little of that assessment. It was very short. Suddenly I was told that I was being detained under section 2 of the Mental Health Act because they believed that I had a mental disorder. I couldn't believe it. I was terrified. Losing my freedom was, at that point, the worst and most frightening thing I could imagine. I had lost control of my own life. I knew that they could treat me with medication or give me other treatments against my will. Having some control of my life was so important. It is a natural response, after a traumatic event (such as I experienced in March of that year) to feel a need to be in control, since you are likely to have lost all sense of control during the traumatic event. That traumatic event came uninvited. It was totally unexpected, happened very suddenly and it was something that I could not ever have imagined. I had no control over what was happening. I couldn't stop it or change it.

The general hospital staff walked with me along the corridor to the vehicle that would transport me to the psychiatric hospital. My thoughts were now on how to escape and I felt that my only option was to run as soon as we walked out of the hospital doors. The staff were clearly expecting this to happen. Very quickly I found myself being held by four members of hospital staff, as soon as I attempted to run. I tried desperately hard to pull away from them. I wouldn't have tried to hurt them in my attempts to secure my freedom, but I did everything that I could to escape from their grasp.

A police car was called to accompany the ambulance in case I attempted to escape again. One of the officers was PC "Smith", the same officer who I had encountered a month earlier. He was the officer who had used physical force and had taken me to the 136 suite. The fact that I had been considered "not detainable" by psychiatrists on that occasion meant that this detention was even more of a shock.

After the struggle with hospital staff at the general hospital, who prevented my attempt to escape before I was transported to the psychiatric hospital, I was placed in the ambulance. I remember searching in my bag for anything that I might be able to use to end my life. I found something that, I felt, could be used, and took it out. It was taken from me by ambulance staff, obviously. I think it perhaps demonstrated my state of mind that I was searching for the means to end my life in full view of ambulance staff. If I had been able to think more clearly, I would have been able to predict that this would only lead to it being removed from me.

As we neared the psychiatric hospital, I asked the ambulance staff "If I swear at a policeman, will I be arrested?" The ambulance staff told me no, I wouldn't be arrested. In retrospect I was, of course, detained under the Mental Health Act and, as such, would not be held accountable.

As I walked up the steps leading to the entrance of the psychiatric hospital, accompanied by the ambulance staff and the police officers, I stopped and turned to PC Smith: "I need to say something. You're a ****ing sadistic ****ard." Before 2012 I never swore. But I think it was perhaps understandable, that night, in my highly emotional state.

I felt it was no coincidence that PC Smith had been the one to respond to the call to attend the hospital. He hadn't been successful in having me detained the previous time and knew he was in trouble over incorrect use of a 136, and his actions in my home.

I was immediately taken to my allocated room on P Ward at the psychiatric hospital. A nurse sat by my bed. I was to be watched 24 hours a day because I was considered particularly high risk. I was told that I would have a member of staff present at all times including when I showered. There was to be no privacy.

Throughout that first night I tried any way I could to end my life.

The following morning, it was clear to staff that I was not going to take food or fluids and I expressed an intention to refuse them, for as long as it took to either kill me, or ensure that I became so unwell that I would have to be taken to a different type of hospital for treatment.

This refusal of food and fluids led to my request to see a psychiatrist being agreed quite quickly. It was a crisis team psychiatrist ("Dr D") who also worked in the psych hospital. He had seen me when I was under the crisis team and knew my case and history. To my absolute shock and relief, he agreed that the psychiatric hospital was not the best place for me. He told me that he was going to discharge me – less than 24 hours after I had been detained under the Mental Health Act. The other staff members in the room were equally shocked. I don't think they knew how to respond. One said: "So we take her off 24 hour watch?" I don't think they could comprehend what was happening. The psychiatrist did tell me that he was "very nervous" about discharging me and that "his job may be on the line" if I died by suicide after being discharged. Well, yes.

I later accessed my psychiatric records and staff documented their concerns about this decision by the psychiatrist.

From my perspective, it was a good decision on the part of the psychiatrist. However, I now question his readiness to discharge me from hospital when I was at high risk of suicide. During subsequent admissions, he showed a willingness to discharge me, when I was still a suicide risk.

While I waited for them to arrange transport home, I went into the communal areas to get something to eat and drink.

The other patients welcomed me and were keen to help. It was a mixed ward and the men, in particular, wanted to assist me. They wanted to make me a drink and show me where the food was stored so that I could get a sandwich. One patient had finished his lunch, but there were still some chips remaining on his plate, and he offered them to me. The patients immediately included me, and showed me acts of kindness.

The other patients didn't realise that I wasn't going to stay and so, from their perspective, I was a new patient. They gave me advice on how best to get through my time there.

The nurses on the ward tried to encourage me to remain at the hospital as an informal patient, and they were clearly concerned that the section had been removed. But I had been taken there against my will and felt that I needed to go home to recover from everything that had happened.

My relief at going home quickly subsided on that first night home. I went into a terrible place emotionally and mentally, and the psychiatrist who discharged me said he felt that I had been re-traumatised by the whole experience of being sectioned and forcibly taken to a place, against my will. The next ten days were horrendous.

The experience of spending a few hours on P Ward, once the section had been lifted, removed much of my fear of psychiatric hospitals, though. Over the next year I had three other psychiatric hospital admissions – each of around a week and all within a twelve month period. I was admitted because I was a suicide risk. It is extremely difficult to get psychiatric hospital admissions, and I was fortunate to be able to do so.

I experienced so much during those three psychiatric hospital admissions, as I will explain later in the book.

It was only just over a month after that substantial overdose that we celebrated the incorporation of Suicide Crisis, when it was set up as a company, and registered as such at Companies

House. As we had set it up to conform to the requirements needed to be recognised as a charity, it was also a charity. I worked extraordinarily long hours in the weeks leading up to registering at Companies House – night after night on the legal aspects, contacting lawyers by email who gave me free advice and looked at all the documents to ensure that everything was done legally correctly. I needed to pay such close attention to detail for the Articles of Association – the very lengthy legal 'rules and regulations' that bound our company and charity. In retrospect, I wonder if I was experiencing a bipolar high during that month, because my behaviour contrasts so markedly with the despair and suicide attempts of November. During a bipolar high (hypomania), I have an extraordinary amount of energy and can work extremely long hours, and am highly productive.

I had a contact (Guy) in a Public Relations company. We needed a website and he was immediately keen to help, offering to create a logo at the same time at a substantially reduced rate.

There was such a sense of excitement in December 2012. We were now officially a company and a charity, and we had a website, a logo, and we started to receive our first donations. Initially our charity was named the Suicide Crisis Centre. However, the logo that was created by Guy and Roger said simply Suicide Crisis. I liked this, and changed the name of our charity to Suicide Crisis a couple of months later. Guy's logic was that we would be wherever the crisis was, so the wording Suicide Crisis was more appropriate and indeed, that proved correct once we set up our services. We attended to people in crisis at many other locations – not just at our Suicide Crisis Centre.

After the exhilaration of December 2012, and our official incorporation, the hard work really began. This was now the preparation phase – working on all aspects of the setting up of the Suicide Crisis Centre and the months of planning, attention to detail, risk assessing, arranging training for our team, finding the right premises and, crucially, finding the right staff, with the right personal qualities.

I visited several properties and buildings before finding premises in the centre of Cheltenham, which provided just what we needed. Its central location meant that it could be accessed easily by people from all parts of Cheltenham and indeed the whole county, as buses came into the centre of Cheltenham from surrounding areas. Our rooms had large windows that looked onto reception, so we could see into them at all times. This was important in terms of minimising risks. There are security cameras covering the entrance, which had large glass doors and an open forecourt, so we could see clearly who was trying to enter. When I first walked into the building to have a look at it, there was an atmosphere of calm and stillness, but it felt very welcoming. I instinctively felt that our clients would feel comfortable here, even before we had done the detailed risk assessments which showed that it was exactly what we were looking for.

Training of staff was going to be hugely important and I identified the skills and qualifications that our team would need. The clients that we were going to work with would be vulnerable and at risk, and we would need appropriately-trained staff. Although our team members all have counselling training, we are not counselling clients. It would not be appropriate to try to provide counselling for clients who may be intensely suicidal. We provide crisis support, but counselling training provides many of the skills that are so important in crisis support. There is further training around assessment of a person's risk of suicide, and suicide intervention skills training, that all staff need to do. They all take a suicide intervention skills course that is recommended by the Department of Health.

It was the personal qualities of our team that would be so vital, though. We needed to find team members who were caring, kind, sensitive, non-judgmental and respectful towards our clients. If they had lived experience of crisis, in the past, then that would be an additional strength.

I knew the importance of a caring and kind approach, when a person is suicidal. Kindness can be immensely powerful, in reaching a person who is at risk. When a person is suicidal, they may consciously or unconsciously detach from the people around them, as part of a preparation to leave this world. When I encountered kindness, it had the power to break through the barriers that I had so carefully constructed around me. It is so difficult not to respond to it. I sometimes encountered this kindness in a nurse at the general hospital, or an on-call GP, and I know how much it can help, when you are at risk.

We found exceptional team members. We found the people that we needed.

It was during this setting up period that I started to become aware of the level of cynicism and doubt that prevailed amongst people of influence in the county, with regard to my intentions. From the perspective of many people, it was astonishing that a mental health patient could even think that she could set up a Suicide Crisis Centre. There was a kind of disparaging wry amusement at my 'ambitions', and I am sure they imagined that I would soon see sense and give up my plans. They saw the label of 'person with mental health issues, recently suicidal' and that was all that defined me, in their eyes. They failed to see that all of us who have mental health issues and have been in crisis are also individuals with our unique qualities, strengths and characteristics.

In January 2013 I met with a Gloucestershire mental health commissioner to look at the possibility of being commissioned to provide services at our Suicide Crisis Centre. During our meeting, I was subjected to some detailed questioning about the treatment that I had been given for my mental health issues and specifically treatment for the trauma that I had experienced in March 2012. It felt intrusive and it was very upsetting. My mental health issues were clearly an issue, from the perspective of the commissioners.

The commissioner said that they would not look at funding Suicide Crisis until we had demonstrated that people were using our services. "Let's see if people use your services." I doubt that he thought people would do so. During the times when we are inundated with clients, and I go for days with virtually no sleep because crises occur at all times of the day and night, I think back to what the commissioner said. Yes, people use our services, Mr Commissioner.

Relying totally on public donations was financially tough, but it was a huge advantage in the early stages. It allowed our services to evolve to meet the needs of our clients. If we had been commissioned, we would have been funded to provide an agreed model. We would have clearly set out how we were going to run the services, and it would have been hard to deviate from that, because it would have been laid down in the contract. It quickly became clear to us that our service could meet the needs of our clients so much more, if we were able to adapt the model and provide exactly what they were telling us that they needed.

Our very first client at our Trauma Centre played a huge role in showing us some of the additional services that we needed to provide. The Trauma Centre opened four months before our Suicide Crisis Centre and started to provide services at the end of May 2013. The Trauma Centre is about early intervention, because I was very aware, from my own experience, that trauma-related conditions such as PTSD can increase a person's risk of suicide. My experience also showed that a person may wait many months for the psychological therapy that NICE guidelines state is the correct treatment for PTSD. If you are unsupported during that period, you are more likely to go into crisis.

The Trauma Centre dealt with smaller numbers than the Suicide Crisis Centre, and it was an excellent way of working on a small scale initially, before the launch of the Crisis Centre in the autumn, which brought much greater numbers.

Our first client was referred to us from mental health services. The psychiatric nurse who referred him described the horrific event that he had witnessed five weeks earlier. She explained that he had been referred for therapy within the NHS secondary psychological services, and so I knew that it would be a wait of several months for him.

Although huge amounts of Government money have been put into talking therapies in primary care, the same is not always true of secondary care psychological services. If you have more complex and enduring mental health diagnoses, or a more complex trauma, and you are considered to be at higher risk of suicide, then you will be referred to secondary mental health psychological services, where there are more experienced psychologists and clinicians. There are only a small number of such experienced psychologists, which leads to long waiting times.

"He needs to talk to someone now," she said. This was our first client, and I asked her if she thought he would prefer to talk to a man or a woman. "He needs to talk to someone now," she said again. When I phoned him immediately afterwards, his distress was very apparent, and it was clear that he would not be able to get to our Trauma Centre. Our outreach work began that day, because I knew that I needed to go out to see him at his home. Our first client showed us that we needed to provide this facility, when clients were too distressed or too unwell or too afraid to leave their homes.

Our first client was also the reason why I fought so hard to set up a PTSD support group for our clients. I had the idea to do it, but our charity's advising psychiatrist felt that it was too dangerous because of the risk of group members being re-traumatised by hearing other people's trauma. "But what if we make it a rule that group members don't talk about the detail of their trauma?" I asked. "They will anyway. You won't be able to stop them," she replied.

Our first client was desperate to be able to attend the PTSD group that we had been planning. It was very important to him. So I knew that I had to find a way to do it. Over the course of a few days I came up with the idea of group meetings organised around guest speakers. A different speaker would come to each meeting to talk about an aspect of PTSD. This would allow group members to learn about the condition and understand it better. The focus would be on the speaker and not on the group members. I spoke to V, one of our other advisers and she agreed with the model, and re-defined it as a group with an educational purpose. Our advising psychiatrist agreed that we could run it.

Our first client doesn't know the role that he played in the creation of that group. But it wouldn't exist if it hadn't been so important to him. I wouldn't have fought so hard to ensure that it was set up. His trauma was so severe. The group mattered so much to him.

What is particularly interesting is that the group meetings evolved to include more participation from group members. We made very clear the ground rule of not talking about the graphic details of your particular trauma – and that we would need to stop anyone who started to do so. And they proved the psychiatrist wrong. They immediately understood why talking in detail about your trauma could be harmful or triggering to someone else, and agreed the rule. They were concerned about other members of the group, and cared about them, and their response was to be protective of other members.

I became aware from my own experience, as a person with mental health issues setting up a charity, that professionals will often underestimate us. The psychiatrist's assumption was that group members could not be trusted (not to talk about the detail of their trauma). That assumption proved to be incorrect. There often seems to be an unwillingness, or inability, on the part of clinicians and professionals, to trust that people with mental health issues will conduct themselves well – or will put the interests of other people first. One of the things that is so obvious to me is that our clients and group members care about and consider the needs of other people so much.

Our advising psychiatrist was exceptionally helpful to Suicide Crisis, though. She was drawn to the ethos of our charity and, having recently taken early retirement, it was an interesting charity to be involved in, from her perspective.

However, the response from her professional contacts to her involvement in our charity was also interesting. Apparently a very senior person in the Clinical Commissioning Group had been quite incredulous that she was involved in advising our charity. The commissioner had expressed this to our advising psychiatrist, along with her scepticism that I could set up a Suicide Crisis Centre. The person had never met me and was clearly making assumptions, based on the scant knowledge that she had of me – that I was a person with mental health issues, who had recently been suicidal. That information was out there, in the public domain. Her reaction seemed to be one of astonishment that a respectable, apparently sensible psychiatrist could be in any way involved in the charity that was being run by the mental health patient.

The resistance seemed pretty widespread from the 'people of influence'. There is a county suicide prevention forum, designed to bring people together who are working in the field of suicide prevention. As well as local mental health services and the police, there were a number of local charities represented on it, some of which had no direct remit to work with people at risk of suicide. However the forum had a relevance to their work, so I understand why it would be helpful for them to be included. In the summer of 2013 we asked for Suicide Crisis to become a member and have a presence at all the forum meetings. The senior Public Health officials, who run it, turned us down. We couldn't understand this at all. I had attended a couple of their meetings as a guest, had been quiet and polite and when I did speak (and I spoke rarely, because I was a little apprehensive, in those early days) it was to say something positive about other services in the county that were being discussed.

It was upsetting to be excluded – and it seemed both incomprehensible and bizarre. We are the one charity in the county that focuses totally on the issue of suicide – and yet we were not to be part of it.

Their explanation was that only our Trauma Centre was open in the summer of 2013. Our Suicide Crisis Centre had not yet opened.

My reply was that the Trauma Centre was about early intervention – supporting people before they reach crisis point, because trauma-related conditions such as PTSD are known to raise the risk of suicide in some people. The Trauma Centre is about helping to prevent suicide. I referred the senior public health official to the county suicide prevention strategy that she oversaw – where veterans with PTSD were named as a group of people who needed to be particularly focused upon, in terms of trying to reduce the number of suicides in the county. Her reason for excluding us made no sense, and only contributed to the feeling that our charity was being discriminated against.

The lack of support and the resistance made things very hard – both practically and emotionally. It definitely impacted upon me emotionally. In order to continue, you have to be extraordinarily passionate about your work, and believe in it when the voices around you are telling you that you (a mental health patient) can't possibly do this.

As well as battling against the forces of scepticism in the county, I was facing my own internal battles. As the months passed, it became clear that the horrific incident in March 2012 had triggered memories of previous trauma, which had been locked away in my mind until then. I was now having flashbacks of this, as well as the incident in 2012. It felt as if the previous trauma had happened in 2012, along with the more recent trauma, because it was so vivid and I remembered it in such detail. The psychological impact and implications felt too much to bear.

I have lost count of the number of different reasons they have given, at various points, for not providing me with the psychological therapy that NICE guidelines state is the appropriate treatment for PTSD. Even when I had the PTSD diagnosis in July 2013, I was not provided with trauma-focused therapy. One of the reasons given was that therapy would raise my suicide risk. Our advising psychiatrist was becoming increasingly concerned about me in the late summer and she wrote to my local mental health trust. She was witnessing my having flashbacks, and she wrote that she felt that I could "do the work" that therapy involved. Nothing happened, though.

My internal life was increasingly a kind of mental hell. It became unbearable to live like this, with no prospect of the therapy that might help. Their withholding of therapy also led to a profound sense of powerlessness and loss of control. They had total control over whether I had therapy or not. And they chose not to provide it.

Suicide seemed the only escape from my inner turmoil. It seemed the only way I could stop it. I had no control over my symptoms and no way of stopping them. Flashbacks and nightmares - those constant dark reminders of past events - arrived uninvited. And the psychological impact of what had happened, what I had experienced – none of that had been addressed by clinicians.

A few weeks earlier there had been a newspaper article about the suicide of a couple. The newspaper article referred to a book where they had obtained the information to end their life. The newspaper did not name the book, but there was enough information to allow me to do an internet search which took me directly to a website where the book was on sale. I ordered it, read it carefully and set about the process of accessing the suicide method. It was an unusual, little known suicide method, but it was highly effective, according to the manual that I had purchased. It was unlikely to fail. Obtaining the suicide method was not easy, and I went to great lengths to obtain it. This is what later made clinicians particularly concerned – the determination with which I acted to obtain it. I have obtained my psychiatric records and the psychiatrist entries confirm that it is a lethal method, if the correct quantity is used.

So in October, I obtained a lethal method to end my life. A week before my intended suicide date, I wrote to my local mental health trust stating very clearly my suicide plan, describing my chosen method, how I had obtained it, and my intention to use it on the following Saturday. I explained my reason was that I could no longer live with the effects of trauma.

For so long I had felt controlled by mental health services. They were able to withhold the one thing that I thought might help me – psychological therapy. I had never been involved in my care plans. Clinicians went away and had meetings, made decisions and wrote to me or told me their decisions about my care. Suddenly the power balance had changed. Having felt powerless for so long I, at last, had some control. I had let them know that I was going to kill myself on a specified date, and there was nothing they could do about it. I felt that this freed me from their control. They could not prevent me from ending my life, which meant that they were no longer in control of me. In retrospect, this thought process suggested I was quite unwell.

As the week went on I remember that I felt less in control – that my death was something that had to happen. I remember feeling at one point that there was a perfect balance of power –

none of us had the power any more. The mental health trust didn't and I didn't. I remember writing again to the Trust to confirm this, and that I felt this was how it should be.

My psychiatric records show that the Trust believed there was a real risk I would do this. I was not a person to make idle threats.

In the moments before my planned suicide attempt, on the Saturday, I hesitated. It was the thought of my charity that caused me to hesitate. I phoned the crisis team and asked for psychiatric hospital admission. It happened very quickly. They arrived at my home twenty minutes later to take me to the psychiatric unit. They were aware of the current risk.

That hospital admission seemed to help initially. I was on 15-minute suicide watch for several days and was only allowed to leave the hospital if I was accompanied by a member of staff. Although this was very restrictive, the nurses assigned to me tried to ensure that the contact with them was therapeutic and not intrusive. Some of the nurses on A Ward were extremely dedicated and skilled. There were three nurses, in particular, who were assigned to my case, with whom I engaged well. They were empathic, caring and supportive, and treated patients with respect and compassion.

They tried to accommodate the individual needs of each patient. In my case, they tried to accommodate the difficulties I was experiencing over food. During the traumatic events, I had no control over what happened. I felt a profound sense of powerlessness. In the months that followed, I struggled to find areas of my life that I could control. My weight became a focus. This was something that I felt I could control, and I became intent on remaining the same weight. If I put on a couple of pounds, it was frightening, because I felt that my weight would quickly spiral out of control. An increase of a couple of pounds necessitated an immediate reduction in the amount of food that I ate, in order to return to the original weight. This had nothing to do with vanity or a focus on appearance. It was motivated by fear, and an attempt to perhaps try to impose some kind of order and control in a world that felt increasingly chaotic, uncertain and unsafe.

I feared the hospital food. I had no idea of its calorie content or the impact that it might have upon my weight. In discussions with ward staff, I asked for permission to buy and prepare my own food, and it was agreed that a member of staff would accompany me to a local supermarket so that I could buy food. I was also allowed to weigh myself every day, because I would have found it difficult to eat if I did not know my current weight.

I got to know some of the other patients, most of whom were detained under the Mental Health Act. It was a mixed ward and I remember one of the male patients on the ward coming up to me on the first night and saying "Don't worry. You'll be okay. I'll be looking out for you. I won't let anything happen to you." He knew it was my first real psych hospital admission and I was nervous.

I liked the other patients on A Ward. There was a very strong, maternal female patient who welcomed all new patients who came to the ward. She was the mother figure. The man who had reassured me on the first night was her partner. They met and started their relationship on the ward.

The only concerning incident was early one morning when I was in the kitchen and a male patient came up behind me and stroked my hair, from the top of my head to the ends of my hair, as if I were a cat. I turned round to look at him, and he smiled at me. It was unsettling, and it felt invasive, but I was not afraid.

I was quiet on the ward but I would not allow myself to be bullied. There was another strong female on the ward and I heard her doing an impersonation of me in one of the communal areas. I walked up to her and said "Hi. I think you just did an impersonation of me." She looked totally surprised and denied it. I calmly told her that I felt sure that she had, and quoted what she had said. At this point a couple of nurses came up to us (presumably fearing that a fight was going to take place). But I was very calm. That incident was helpful. No one impersonated me or tried to belittle me after that.

By the Thursday, I was very low and intent on suicide. I asked to discharge myself, but the ward psychiatrist said he needed to seek a second opinion on whether I should be assessed under the Mental Health Act (MHA), with a view to sectioning me. He told me that he felt that, if he allowed me to leave on the Thursday, he would be sending me home to "certain death". This related to the suicide method that he knew I had obtained.

Initially I understood his wish to get a second opinion. I recognised the weight that he would carry, making a decision, alone, which might lead to the death of a patient.

However, the ward staff gave me no information over the next 24 hours about whether I was about to be assessed under the Mental Health Act or not. The prospect of being sectioned was very frightening for me and I repeatedly asked what was happening, only to be met with responses that seemed evasive. Eventually I was told that I needed to wait to see the psychiatrist. From that point, they referred to the meeting as being with a single psychiatrist. That was reassuring. A single psychiatrist meant that it would not be a Mental Health Act assessment.

I walked into the room, expecting to see one psychiatrist, and saw four people. I immediately knew this was a Mental Health Act assessment. I felt a mixture of fear, shock and anger. Anger was what came out initially.

There was a point in the assessment where I became very fearful that I would be detained. However, I think my display of anger at the beginning of the meeting helped me. The psychiatrist was, I think, more reassured to see an angry person, who was effectively still fighting, than the subdued person, that he had seen the previous day, who had given up.

However, I was fighting for my freedom – not for my life.

As soon as they told me that they would not be detaining me, I asked to leave.

What they failed to pick up, in the assessment, was that I still had a very strong intent to end my life. That had not diminished. In the MHA assessment, all my energies had been focused on not being detained. That energy burst seemed to reassure them. Once it was over, the anger, stress and shock that I felt, over the unexpected MHA assessment, added to my suicidal intent. Anger can raise a person's risk of suicide. That is well documented.

I arrived home, walked in, let my coat fall on the floor and walked into the dining room to write a suicide note. I was fully intent on suicide and had the lethal method upstairs. I was still so angry and the note reflected that. I read it back and knew that this was not the note that I wanted to leave behind. This note did not reflect what I would have wanted to write. I felt that, if I waited an hour, I might be calmer and could write a note that would provide some explanation and perhaps comfort, rather than the current note, which was accusatory toward mental health services. The waiting prevented the suicide attempt. It was anger that was fuelling the sense of urgency to end my life. By waiting, in order to write a more considered final note to leave behind, it meant that my rage dissipated. As my anger diminished, the sense of imminent need to end my life gradually subsided. I was still feeling suicidal, but the factors fuelling an imminent attempt had been reduced. I was able to stay safe that night and in the days that followed.

It's important to be aware that anger can raise the risk of suicide. I have seen this in our clients, where a sudden outburst of rage is fuelling suicidal intent and making the prospect of an imminent attempt very real. We often experience this via our emergency phone line when a known client has experienced something that has been inflammatory. Talking to someone who understands why you are angry, and who can help you to work through it, can massively reduce the immediate risk.

During my psychiatric hospital admission I had been picking up phone messages from the media who were aware that the opening of our Suicide Crisis Centre was in mid-

October. Our media director told them I was "unwell" but gave no details. I was aware that there was probably a bigger story for them, in that the founder of the charity was an inpatient in a psychiatric hospital and was herself a suicide risk.

A few days later I was doing a round of media interviews for press, radio and TV for the opening of our Suicide Crisis Centre. That was incredibly hard, so soon after discharge. Days later our crisis centre opened and we were inundated with clients. I went straight from psychiatric hospital to all this.

Those first few months were incredibly busy. It was the run-up to Christmas. It was so rewarding, though. We knew that the centre was making a difference and that we were helping people.

It had been very important to me that we would be open on Christmas Day.

In those first few months the majority of our clients were not accessing other services. They were exactly the kind of clients that we wanted to reach – people who would not go to their GP or phone other services, and whose silence about their suicidality put them at risk. As the months went on, we were increasingly being accessed by people who were under the care of mental health services, but were not finding that support sufficient. Sometimes they were just not finding it helpful. We were being accessed by people under secondary mental health services who had more complex and long-standing mental health issues. It was distressing to see how many of them could not access NHS psychological therapy, or found the crisis team unhelpful and would not use them.

I was able to work productively for several months, because the work and the clients gave me a purpose. I cared very much about them and their survival was very, very important to me. I remember talking to a colleague about one of our clients who was particularly high risk, and breaking down in tears, because I felt there was a very real risk that he would die. We get to know our clients well and that is the result – the death of a client has a profound effect. Even the prospect of their death can feel painful. This client didn't die, to our great joy and relief, but, several months later, a former client did die whilst under the care of mental health services, and it was devastating. I'll tell you about Juliet later. I still find it painful to talk about Juliet's death.

The workload in those first six months was huge and it was a seven-day a week commitment. By April I was exhausted and very low, and I was admitted to psychiatric hospital because I was considered to be a suicide risk again. Bipolar had still not been diagnosed, so no one was seeing a reason why I was repeatedly going into deep suicidal lows.

My second admission to psychiatric hospital was, in some ways, more eventful than my previous admission in October 2013. It was during this April admission that I escaped, whilst detained under a section 5.2 at the psychiatric hospital.

When I was admitted in April, it was once again because of suicide risk. I was admitted as an informal (voluntary) patient - this time to a female ward. On the day I was admitted I was assessed as being at high risk of suicide, according to my care plan of 23rd April.

However, on 24th April, Dr D revised the care plan, lowering the risk to medium, writing:-

"Should Joy wish to leave hospital, this should be agreed, even if she is voicing suicidal ideation / intent."

It was a shock to read this. I couldn't believe that a psychiatrist would actually write this on a care plan. It appeared that no one would even attempt to talk to me about my plan to kill myself, if I discharged myself from hospital, stating an intention to end my life. Despite the fact that I was an informal patient, I would have believed that there was some duty of care on the part of the psychiatrist and the hospital to ensure I was assessed before leaving, if I was expressing suicidal intent.

A friend of mine, who is a psychiatric nurse in another part of the country, wrote to the psychiatric hospital to express her concern about this entry on the care plan. She gave her opinion that a nurse's registration may be affected if they allowed me to walk out of hospital, stating an intention to kill myself. She felt it was tantamount to allowing or assisting a suicide. This made some of the nurses nervous, I think, and, when I became highly distressed mid-week and stated an intention to leave hospital, when I was clearly suicidal, the first nurse that I spoke to asked me to wait until her shift had finished. I didn't realise why at the time – I thought they wanted me to wait and have time to think, but, in retrospect, I think she was nervous about her own position, if she had been the one who allowed me to leave.

The nurses spoke during their handover meeting at the end of the shift and asked the duty psychiatrist to assess me. I remember that I was having some difficulty thinking clearly and expressing myself, because I was very distressed. As a result of my apparent lack of clarity of thought, the duty psychiatrist put me under a section 5.2. This is a 72-hour section which leads to a full assessment under the Mental Health Act.

Being detained was always a difficult and frightening experience for me. Up until then I had had a certain amount of freedom to leave the hospital to go to the shops, or go for a walk. Now I felt contained, imprisoned – and I was extremely fearful that the MHA assessment might lead to longer detention.

The feeling of being imprisoned was unbearable and I felt an overwhelming need to escape.

Just after 9.30pm one of the patients became extremely agitated and started shouting very loudly. She was in her room at the end of the corridor, and all the ward staff rushed down to her. There are very few staff on duty from 9.30pm. Far fewer than in the daytime.

I was in the communal area near the exit door of the ward. The only other people left in the communal area were two patients who were sitting on the floor. They had been talking but fell silent. I turned to look at them briefly and they looked back at me. I hesitated a moment, and then turned and walked quickly out of the ward door. I had obviously been seen leaving and I knew that it was likely they would inform staff, so I had to be very, very quick. I ran down the stairs to the main entrance. I knew that the main doors would be locked at 10pm. I encountered no one – I did not even see a receptionist – and I ran out of the main door and down the road. I was still in the hospital complex initially, because the psychiatric hospital is in the same area as the general hospital. In my panic, I turned right too early and found myself in a car park. I quickly ran back and then found the correct exit onto London Road. Now I was free, but on a main road and easily seen, so I continued to run until I reached some side roads.

This was the point where I felt a massive sense of euphoria. I really was free, and remember calling a friend to express my delight, describing the beautiful starry night to him. He was frightened. "Joy, you have to go back," he said. He was obviously fearful for my safety – not just my suicide risk but also the fact that I was a lone female out on the streets. None of this occurred to me, in my euphoric state.

I realised that I was nearing Gloucester Park. I had lived with my nan in the first few years of my life, right by Gloucester Park. It was a place of good memories for me. So I went to look at Gloucester Park. Then I thought of the cathedral. That was beautiful. I needed to go and look at Gloucester Cathedral. I was, in effect, doing a sightseeing tour of Gloucester. After the cathedral, I walked through the town centre. I walked past a pub where there was live music. A female singer had a captivating voice and I stopped outside the pub to listen. A man invited me in – I think he may have been the owner.

So I went into the pub, and was made welcome by the regulars. I was a sectioned mental health patient who had escaped from psychiatric hospital, and was now enjoying a drink with the regulars in a friendly Gloucester pub. I wondered what the pub regulars would have thought, if they knew the reality of my situation.

I was aware that my phone was ringing quite a lot. It was the hospital ward, leaving messages asking me to return immediately. Psychiatric hospital under section – or pub? You can see the dilemma.

I enjoyed the relaxed, friendly atmosphere for some time, but eventually it was time to leave. What to do now? The police would have been alerted by now.

I walked and reflected upon my situation. I was starting to realise that, if I continued to run, it would soon be reported in the newspapers – a missing person who was vulnerable. I thought about the effect upon our charity. And where could I run to? I couldn't run indefinitely. It felt as if the only option was to return. I walked back to the hospital, and saw a police van outside. I rang the bell and was let in. It seemed so incongruous – calmly ringing the bell to get back in, after my escape. The nurses on the ward expressed their anger. I think perhaps they don't realise how frightening it is to be sectioned and how you experience a total loss of freedom, power and control over your own life.

I went into the kitchen and the two patients who had seen me leaving were in the adjoining dining room.

One of them looked at me, paused, and then said:-

"Well, I didn't expect that of Olivia Newton John over there".

I was assessed under the Mental Health Act the next day. I said little and was clearly depressed, but was allowed to discharge myself. I was not voicing suicidal intent.

Despite the difficulties that I encountered, there were positive aspects of my first two stays in psychiatric hospital. During my first admission to A Ward, in particular, I encountered staff members who were dedicated and clearly wanted to help to ensure that the admission was therapeutic. I cannot say the same about my third admission to psychiatric hospital, which was to a different ward.

It was the first week of September 2014. That was the stay that led to my decision never to access mental health care again in this county. Some of the things that staff members said to me, during that admission, should never be said to anyone, particularly a person in a psychiatric hospital, who is clearly vulnerable.

My admission was triggered, once again, by a loss of hope over accessing appropriate therapy for trauma.

After the October 2013 hospital admission, I was offered some therapy with Dr C, but it was not trauma-focused therapy. The sessions appeared unstructured and involved long periods sitting in silence. I had no idea what I should say, or what was expected of me. These long silences were profoundly unsettling. I felt lost in a vast open space, where there is nothing safe. It was the opposite of helpful, for a person who had experienced trauma. My friend who works in psychiatric services wrote to my mental health trust to express her concern that this type of therapy could increase my risks. After three sessions, I stopped attending the appointments. One of the Oxford psychiatrists told me this year that it sounded like psychoanalytical therapy, and he felt that this was not what I needed.

A few weeks after I stopped attending the sessions, I arranged a meeting with my local mental health trust to request trauma-focused therapy. Their medical director agreed that they would arrange this, and an email from the Trust confirmed they would arrange for me to see another therapist. It never happened. Dr C, who had provided the therapy, stated that he felt my disengagement was an indication that I could not engage in a therapeutic relationship. I was clearly "not ready" for therapy, in his view. He was a very senior clinician, and his view overruled the management decision to provide trauma-focused therapy. It was devastating. I disengaged because the therapy was inappropriate for a person with a diagnosis of PTSD, not because I was unable to engage in a therapeutic relationship. I had issues of trust, but these should not have been considered insurmountable.

In the weeks leading up to my third admission to psychiatric hospital, I had contact with a mental health team in Gloucestershire. They told me that it would be another year to eighteen months before I would even be considered for therapy. I was extremely distressed and phoned Dr D directly, asking if this was his decision. He told me that Dr C had made the decision, on the grounds that I hadn't demonstrated that I could build a therapeutic relationship with a mental health professional. In eighteen months' time, it would be four years since I first asked for psychological therapy. It is stated often in my psychiatric records that psychological therapy is 'the treatment of choice' for me. And yet I could never access the trauma-focused treatment that would be the most appropriate for me. Four years. And even then it would only be 'considered'.

It seems inhumane to me that a person, who has been through extremely traumatic events, would be left without appropriate treatment for four years or more.

A traumatic event propelled me into this crisis, and into this mental health land, and I have never been able to come out of it. The bipolar diagnosis means that I will never leave mental health land. I know that. But I am also locked in my own post-traumatic world, from which there is no apparent escape. Both the Oxford psychiatrists who assessed me in 2015 felt psychological therapy was needed specifically for trauma.

Surely an accomplished psychological therapist would understand that it is not unusual for a person who has been through trauma to find it difficult to trust, since their whole world view may have been shattered in a matter of minutes, during the traumatic event. Their perception of the world as a relatively safe place may have gone. Their trust in other people may have evaporated. That person may, therefore, find it difficult to build a trusting relationship with a therapist – but that would surely be part of the work of the therapist to work to help that person to engage with them in the early stages, before intensive therapy begins.

A wait of at least another eighteen months for therapy meant eighteen more months of the torturous life I was leading – a life where I worked seventeen hour days so I didn't have to think. Avoidance is a classic PTSD trait. I'm an expert in it. Working excessively and intensively blocks out the past traumas that relentlessly seek to seep into my consciousness.

To live another eighteen months like that was unimaginable. It felt unbearable. I was intent on suicide to exit from a life that felt intolerable.

I requested psychiatric hospital admission from the crisis team. They were reluctant to provide it initially but I made clear my suicidal intent. They discussed the situation with the duty psychiatrist and he said that I should be offered a week's "respite stay" in the psychiatric hospital. This was a new plan that Dr D had created recently. I had no input into this care plan. It was decided by mental health professionals, without consulting me at all. This was what always happened. Clinicians had meetings and discussions, then informed me of the outcome of those meetings and discussions and presented me with my treatment plan. Patients are supposed to be consulted, but I never have been. I was to be offered three respite admissions a year. The crisis team advised me that these respite admissions of a week's duration were to be used before I reached crisis point and were a means of preventing me from going into crisis. "But I am already in crisis. I attempted suicide last night," I said.

I was told that it could not be an acute psychiatric admission. In my case, the psychiatric hospital would only be for respite. When at risk of suicide, I was to be supported by the mental health team in the community. So, in order for me to be admitted to psychiatric hospital, I had to say that I would accept a 'respite stay', despite being in crisis. If you attempt suicide, using a violent method that you have previously stated that you could never imagine using, then this would suggest that you are in crisis.

Initially I was admitted to P Ward, which is a mixed ward. I was highly distressed and repeatedly asked to leave, with the intention of ending my life. I wouldn't guarantee my safety on leaving. I was considered by the duty psychiatrists to be detainable and was told that, if I tried to leave, I would be put under a section 5.2. Nurses had already been putting me under section 5.4s. One of the duty psychiatrists said to me "This feels more like a crisis admission than a respite admission." I think it should have been obvious from the start that it should have been a crisis admission but Dr D (and the crisis team) had insisted on adhering to the "plan" - and crisis admission did not form part of that plan. Admissions were for 'respite' - even if you were evidently in crisis.

On Monday Dr D was back and made it clear to the psychiatrists who had detained me that this was a respite stay. I saw him on that day and spoke about my loss of hope over psychological therapy and asked if I could be assessed by a psychologist in the psychiatric hospital, for a second opinion about whether I was ready for psychological therapy. He told me that would not be possible "because that's not what this admission is for. This is a respite admission."

What was very strange, in retrospect, was that he appeared to be very aware of my suicidal feelings and intent, but he was insisting, despite this, that it was to be designated a respite stay.

He said: "It feels like you have reached the end." That is a pretty clear indication that he was aware that I had reached a point where I had no resources left. In saying that, he must have been aware of my risk. I cannot understand why he did not arrange the psychological assessment that I had asked for.

It would not have been difficult to do and, if he was aware that I had "reached the end" and was also aware that the loss of hope revolved around the prospect of never being released from the effects of trauma, then there was something that he could have done, at that point.

By saying "It feels like you have reached the end", it reinforced my sense that this was the end.

He didn't challenge the view that I was at the end, and, indeed, he went on to say "It all sounds hopeless." In retrospect, I wonder why he didn't say "It sounds as if you have lost hope." This would have suggested the patient's loss of hope, rather than reaffirming the patient's belief that things were hopeless – that there was no hope.

As this was a respite stay, I was free to leave the hospital whenever I wished. I went home that afternoon and collected the medication that I had stored there.

Before returning to the psychiatric hospital, I sat for a while on a grass verge opposite it. A male patient, who I had met previously in the hospital courtyard, came over to me and sat beside me. He was an intelligent man who spoke softly, and who appeared quite gentle and calm. However, he would gaze at me quite intently as he spoke. We talked for a while, and then the conservation suddenly altered. He revealed that he had killed a domestic animal in an extremely violent way. He expressed no remorse and indeed became aggressive as he described what he had done, which he felt was fully justified. I was deeply shocked.

That evening I went out into the hospital courtyard. A friend on the outside had asked me to go out and look at the moon, which was particularly beautiful that night, he said. One of the male patients from P ward came out and hugged me, prompting a reprimand from the nurse who accompanied him. She stood by the door to the courtyard while he and I sat on a bench. There was a massive moon that evening – it was extraordinary. He turned to me and told me that he loved me. He then went on to tell me that he would demonstrate to me that he loved me. I wasn't totally sure what was happening here, and asked what he meant. He then moved close to me and described the way in which he would physically demonstrate his love for me by having sex with me.

The nurse called to him that it was time to go back to the ward.

I looked at the moon for a final time and went upstairs. A nurse on the ward asked me how my day had been. "Terrible" I replied. She simply said "Oh" and didn't seek to explore further.

I went to my room shortly after 10pm. The nurses are supposed to check patients every hour at night but they missed the next check, in my case.

One of the things that I have never understood is the lack of checks on patients at night. Even when I was on 15-minute suicide watch in the daytime, during my first psychiatric hospital admission on 2013, the checks were only hourly at night. This is presumably because there are far fewer staff members at night, but in terms of patient safety, it is extremely concerning.

Although my intention, earlier in the day, had been to use medication to end my life, I attempted suicide using a method which was quicker and more immediate. There had been a well-publicised suicide of a celebrity recently, and there was some very detailed information on the internet about the method that he had used, which I had remembered.

I was found by a nursing assistant who came into my room, and who raised the alert which led to a colleague arriving. She detached me, and then threw me face down on the bed. I wasn't sure what was happening and was confused and frightened. It felt as if she hit me several times on the head but it may have been an attempt to remove my suicide method. She didn't speak at all and I think that is what made it more frightening.

She left the room, still having said nothing. Shortly afterwards a colleague of hers came in. She said to me:-

"If you want to kill yourself, do it at home. Don't come into hospital to do it. You're an informal patient."

It was profoundly shocking, and extremely distressing, to hear that. When I later raised this incident formally with the mental health trust and the NMC, the nurse denied having said it, and there were no witnesses to it. This meant that my complaint could not be progressed, as a result of her and my conflicting evidence, and the lack of witnesses.

She said it. I am absolutely certain of my recollection of this incident. I recall her exact words, precisely because it was so shocking to hear a psychiatric nurse say this. Her words are imprinted upon my mind. She may have been under extreme stress, and may have been reacting out of anger induced by the shock of a suicide attempt "on her watch", but it was a highly dangerous, irresponsible comment on her part. It showed not just a total lack of compassion, but also a total lack of understanding of suicidal behaviour, and the frame of mind that a person is in, when they attempt suicide.

It was such an extraordinarily uncaring comment. At the point where you are at your most vulnerable, when you are already in such deep emotional pain, that you want to extinguish your own life, you encounter a response that increases your pain. Not only do staff not appear to care whether you live or die, they are now suggesting that, if you want to die, that you do it in a place which is less inconvenient to them. It is not difficult to see why her comment only increased my suicidal intent. My immediate thought was that I would go home and kill myself and I asked to leave at once. I wasn't allowed to leave and was put under a section (a nurse's holding power) overnight.

I attempted to phone my friend, Tim, because I desperately needed to talk to someone. The same nurse prevented this, saying: "Your friend will have better things to do than talk to you."

It was such an unkind remark. The message was that I mattered so little, that a friend would not wish to allocate any time to me, even when I had made a suicide attempt and still felt that I wanted to die. The message was that my life had no value. I already felt this. Most of us, who are depressed and contemplating suicide, believe this. Her words simply reinforced the feeling.

My friend was furious at her comment. He said there could have been nothing more important than talking to his friend, who was suicidal, that night. He subsequently raised a formal complaint with our local mental health service, in which he wrote:-

"I find it outrageous that any member of your staff should presume to tell my friend how much or how little I care about her."

The duty psychiatrist came in early the next morning and assessed that I had the mental capacity to make decisions, which meant that I was allowed to leave. Dr D's directive of April 2013 continued to be applied. It was on record that I should be allowed to leave, even if expressing suicidal intent. One of the nurses asked me to stay until Dr D came on duty at 9am, since she felt that he may feel differently about the directive that he had issued, after the suicide attempt in hospital. However, he agreed that I should be allowed to leave, realising, I believe, that this had been a disastrous admission, which was providing nothing therapeutic for me and which was increasing my suicide risk, rather than diminishing it.

If the admission had been treated as a crisis admission, and I had received appropriate support for a person who was in crisis, then it could, perhaps, have been a therapeutic admission.

I left the hospital without even taking my belongings. All my clothes were still there. I simply walked out. I reached Gloucester city centre and broke down. I sat on the pavement, crying. I recall a woman stopping to ask me if I was okay but I was too distressed to even answer. Sometime afterwards I was aware that someone was saying my name "Joy". I looked up and saw a woman who I knew professionally, in the context of my work. It was pure chance that she had walked by. I went to sit with her on a nearby bench and told her that I had just left psychiatric hospital. She wasn't sure what to do but she was married to a psychiatrist and she called him. I could not hear his questions but she gave our location in the city centre and I knew that meant that he would be calling the police. I immediately stood up, and told her that I would have to go. She stood up, too. I hugged her and said that I was sorry. I was surprised to see tears in her eyes. I left quickly because I knew that the police had probably already been called by her husband.

I walked quickly away from the city centre and headed for the docks. As I approached the docks, I turned and thought I could see the woman following me. This was alarming as it meant she could inform police where I was. I started to run. I turned into an arcade but, as I did so, I heard a man shout out my name and I realised that the police were following me. I knew I had the medication in my bag and I was terrified that they would take it. I ran into some ladies' toilets and quickly entered a cubicle, locking the door behind me. The police moved very fast and the policeman was over the top of the cubicle within seconds.

The policeman and his female colleague took me outside and we sat on a bench. The woman had caught up with us and she joined us. She looked hesitant, as she approached, and I think she expected me to be angry with her. I wasn't. I would have done the same, if it had been her. I understood.

It was clear that the police were going to detain me under a section 136. I wasn't prepared to go back to the psychiatric hospital voluntarily. They were pleasant, though, which isn't always the case with police officers who are called to people who are a suicide risk.

During the Mental Health Act assessment at the 136 suite, I thought I might be detained, at one point. I had said that I had no plans to go home and intended to stay on the streets of Gloucester. I couldn't bear the idea of going home. I think that made the female psychiatrist concerned about the safety of a lone female out on the streets all night, who had just discharged herself from psychiatric hospital. However, they didn't detain me and I left the 136 suite. They offered me voluntary admission to the psychiatric hospital, which I refused. I walked out, leaving my clothes and belongings at the hospital.

I spent the night on the streets and that led to some concerning incidents. My ability to judge situations wasn't good. In the early hours of the morning, a lot of men were coming out of pubs. A lone female provoked a certain amount of interest and assumption.

Several of the men offered me a room for the night. One of the men seemed okay and I was cold and thirsty by then, and so I accepted. We walked to the taxi rank but I hesitated as we approached the taxi. He encouraged me to continue and we stood by the taxi as he explained our destination to the driver. Again, I hesitated and he suddenly started to force me into the back of the vehicle. The taxi driver assumed that the man knew me, I think, because he didn't react at all. He seemed to think this was an altercation between a couple. I didn't scream and just focused on extricating myself from him. I struggled free.

However, what surprised me most that night was the number of people who responded with concern, and tried to help.

Two homeless men approached me. They felt that I was potentially vulnerable on the streets, and invited me to come and sleep in the place that they always slept, under a bridge. I was reluctant to do so and they were genuinely worried. "It's not safe for a woman to be out here alone at night." If I wouldn't go with them, then they wanted to leave me a blanket, so that I would be warm. They were kind and they were wise to the dangers of the street. But I was warm enough, I reassured them.

A stranger had also become concerned and he engaged me in conversation, to try to ascertain why I was out on the streets. He was distracted when a person he knew came up to speak to him, and I was gone before he realised it. I heard from the homeless men later that night that the man had been asking about me and was driving around trying to find me. This was extraordinary to me, because I had come from a psychiatric hospital where I hadn't felt there was concern for me – or my life. Here, on the streets, total strangers were trying to help.

A Polish man started talking to me, and he invited me back to his house, where I spent an hour and where his wife gave me hot chocolate and toast.

In retrospect, it's wonderful that there is this level of care and concern. I was born in Gloucester and my family comes from here originally. It makes me feel proud to come from a city where people respond in this way to a person who was clearly vulnerable.

I'm sure this happens elsewhere, too. It's the very best of human nature, isn't it?

Eventually, the police also became concerned about a lone female on the city centre streets in the early hours of the morning, and at around 5am I was taken under a section 136 to the psychiatric hospital.

I recognised the name of one of the psychiatrists who was carrying out the Mental Health Act assessment on that day. He had been treating one of our clients. I remembered that she had described him as 'cold'.

I recall that he said some bizarre things, including "Genuinely suicidal people don't ask for help. They go off quietly and kill themselves." This was extraordinary. He was suggesting that a genuinely suicidal person would not seek help from anyone. A large percentage of people, who have strong suicidal intent, and who may go on to end their lives will, at some point, tell someone or seek help. There is often a small part of them that is trying to survive. This is the part that seeks help. That small part may diminish and that's why it is so vital that we do all we can to help, while we still have an opportunity to do so.

I couldn't understand how a psychiatrist could actually believe something like this – and I said exactly that to him. It seems to me that some mental health clinicians – both nurses and psychiatrists – may have a huge knowledge base about the different mental health conditions. But they seem to have very little real understanding of suicidality. I am told that there is very little focus on it, in training.

They asked me about my experiences overnight on the streets and I told them about some of the incidents, including being forced into the back of a taxi. One of the last things that the psychiatrist said was "If you want to stay out on the streets all night, that's up to you." I think that comment summed up the response from mental health services. Total strangers were concerned about a mentally unwell female on the streets, but mental health services were entirely unconcerned.

During much of my journey through mental health services in my county, I have felt that this lack of concern has been prevalent.

It seems that, if a patient is not detainable, then the responsibilities of mental health services (to the patient) may cease. However, if the patient is suicidal, and particularly if they are mentally unwell, then there is surely still a duty of care towards that patient, even if they are not detainable. Surely there is a duty of care to do all that they can to help a person to survive.

From the perspective of mental health services, there will be no liability for them if the patient kills themselves, if they have mental capacity.

Patients are told directly: "It's your choice" or "It's your decision" to end their life. It was said to me, and our clients are telling us that mental health clinicians are using the same phrase, when they speak to them. It is directed specifically at the patient. The clinicians are not making a general statement: "A person has the choice to end their life". It is being personalised and directed at the individual.

The phrase is presumably being employed to promote individual responsibility.

However, I think that it is a profoundly unhelpful, and possibly dangerous thing to say to a suicidal person who is under the care of mental health services. If you are mentally unwell, and particularly if you are clinically depressed, you are likely to be making a decision that you would not make, if you were well. When depressed, your perceptions, beliefs, interpretation of events and view of the world may be entirely different from usual. Your perspective is altered.

The phrase is being directed at patients who are under secondary mental health services and who, therefore, have more severe and enduring mental health issues. It has been quoted to me by patients who are under secondary mental health services.

I have asked our clients, who are under the care of mental health services and who have been told this, what their reaction has been to it. One client told me: "It makes me feel that they couldn't care less whether I do it." Another client said: "It makes me feel that they want me to do it."

It is obviously not the intention of clinicians that their words should be interpreted in this way. However, this is the risk, when you say it to a person who is mentally unwell, and who may interpret it in a very different way to that which you intend.

I have raised this issue with our local mental health trust. The Trust arranged for me to have a meeting with a senior clinician, who failed to respond directly to the issue that I raised, or explain why that phrase was being used, stating instead that clinicians used many different phrases, when speaking to suicidal people. "Sometimes we say: 'Don't kill yourself' to a patient," he told me. "Do you?" I replied. "When do you say that? Because no client has ever repeated that phrase to me, when they have quoted mental health clinicians." He was not prepared to say under what circumstances they might tell a patient not to kill themself.

When I spoke to the Government's adviser on suicide, I raised the issue with him and he gave his own opinion on it, stating that it would be an example that he could use, to demonstrate what is being said to patients in some parts of the country.

Instead of simply telling patients that it's their choice or their decision to end their life, I wonder why, instead, mental health clinicians don't say: "I want to do what I can to help you to survive."

Suicide Crisis gave a presentation to the Zero Suicide Initiative about our work in early 2015. Zero Suicide was a Government initiative to try to reduce the number of suicides, particularly in NHS patients known to mental health services.

My belief is that zero suicide should mean doing all that we can, for each individual, to help them to survive. That's what Suicide Crisis tries to do. But I do not feel that this is what happens within NHS mental health services currently in this county.

I think back to my care plan for my second stay in psychiatric hospital: "Should Joy wish to leave hospital, this should be agreed, even if she is voicing suicidal ideation/intent." If you are suicidal, you may be able to just walk out of psychiatric hospital and end your life. My final stay in psychiatric hospital demonstrated that. I left that hospital with a lethal dose of medication and an intention to kill myself. The kindness that was shown to me by strangers, on the streets of Gloucester, did more to reduce my suicidal intent than any encounter with a clinician at the psychiatric hospital, during my third admission to hospital.

That admission in September was my final contact with local mental health services. I wanted no more from them after that. I requested my psychiatric records, and the revelations in them cemented my decision to never access their services again. I will never trust them again, after what I read in my records.

In the weeks and months after the September admission, friends and GPs started noticing symptoms that they felt may indicate bipolar. This led to my requesting and being referred (by my GP) for an assessment at a specialist bipolar clinic within Oxford NHS Health Trust. I would not have considered an assessment in my own county, after my recent experience of services here.

In February 2015, the assessing psychiatrist diagnosed bipolar disorder type 2. That means that I experience hypomania, which is less severe than the mania that can be experienced in type one. However, the depressive lows are extreme and it is during those lows that I have been a suicide risk. After a second assessment with a different Oxford psychiatrist in April, he wrote that it may have been the trauma in 2012 that 'uncovered' the bipolar, or allowed it to emerge. I would have had a biological and genetic vulnerability – a relative was diagnosed with bipolar many years ago. He also noted the 'post-traumatic syndrome'. My local mental health trust dropped the diagnosis of PTSD in April 2014. The Oxford psychiatrist reinstated it.

It makes me more sad than I can express that the traumatic event may have uncovered a serious mental health condition – bipolar disorder - that I will have for life. However, it is an explanation of why I have continued to be a suicide risk, at times. It was a diagnosis that went unnoticed until 2015.

I have had a more positive experience of NHS mental health services in Oxford. I have confidence in the specialist services that they provide. There are national centres of excellence in Oxford and their bipolar centre is particularly renowned. I am grateful that my assessments in Oxford led to a correct diagnosis.

Since September 2014 I have made no further suicide attempts. I think my risks have been reduced by a number of factors, the main ones being my bipolar diagnosis, and my self-discharge from local mental health services.

When GPs started to suggest that I might have bipolar, it meant that there was a possible explanation for the depressive lows that I experienced. If my mental health issues were understood, then I could perhaps be helped. It gave me some hope.

The diagnosis this year was initially quite difficult to accept, and I went through a period of denial, but I now acknowledge that I have bipolar. My increased knowledge and understanding of my mental health diagnosis means that I am able to practise self-management of my symptoms, including monitoring my moods and identifying triggers to depressive episodes.

My decision to discharge myself from the care of local mental health services has also helped. I think some aspects of my mental health care increased my suicide risk: the ongoing 'professional puzzlement' of clinicians, the failure to diagnose correctly or to provide relevant treatment (for bipolar, in particular), the withholding of trauma-focused therapy, my lack of involvement in decisions about my care, and the unhelpful responses from some of the individual clinicians.

It is not an approach that I would recommend to most people, though. If a person has a mental health diagnosis, and is able to engage with local services, then local psychiatric services can provide the most immediate sources of support, advice and treatment that should help in the management of the condition. I attend a bipolar support group, which is run by a charity, and many of the group members have had a positive experience of local NHS mental health services.

Those of us who have had negative experiences of mental health services may be profoundly affected by those experiences, though. It is not just the impact of a failure to diagnose correctly, or a lack of appropriate treatment. The greatest harm may be caused by the way that a person is treated by staff.

It is not only in mental health services that patients are encountering inappropriate or unhelpful responses from staff members. It can happen in general hospitals, or in contact with the police, paramedics and GPs. It's important to understand the impact and effect on a person, and on their suicide risk – and to understand how another kind of response, from professionals, could make such a difference, if we are looking at zero suicide as an ambition. It is not that we can realistically prevent all suicides, but if our ambition is that we ensure that all professionals, who come into contact with a suicidal person, act in a way that gives every opportunity for that person to survive, then we may be able to significantly reduce the number of suicides.

We need to be more tenacious in actively helping people to survive. I wish that we could try to create a culture where general hospital staff, police officers and paramedics ensure that they treat every suicidal person with respect, kindness and care. The impact upon a person's suicide risk could be significant, as I will explain after the example that I give of my own experience within a general hospital, after a suicide attempt. I think that a fundamental change in training may be required, so that it includes a focus upon understanding suicidality, the possible reasons why a person may become suicidal, and also allows an exploration of the very complex feelings and attitudes that professionals may have towards patients who present as suicidal, or who have attempted suicide. There is an issue of attitude, amongst some members of staff, towards suicidal people. This needs to be explored in a supportive environment.

Although there are some exceptionally caring nurses within the NHS, who treat suicidal patients with compassion, there are also those who respond extremely negatively to them. They fail to understand or empathise and may see the suicidal patient as taking a bed that could be given to a patient with a physical condition. For some, suicidal intent or attempts provoke anger. I remember encountering anger in a friend, when she became aware that I was suicidal in 2012. She had experienced extremely difficult events, but had never become suicidal. If she had been able to battle through, then why couldn't I, she felt. I think some nurses have that inability to understand, too.

In the spring of 2013, I was hospitalised after taking an overdose of a highly toxic drug. In the hours that followed, I felt as if I was being tortured. I am not sure whether it was the drug itself or the antidote that was so excruciating. But I remember thinking that I did not know how I could survive 60 seconds of this. I was told that I had another 12 hours on the intravenous antidote. It was impossible. My bed was at the end of the ward and I looked up at the open window. It was far too high to reach, but I remember wishing desperately that I could jump from that window. I would have tried anything at that point to escape the physical and mental pain that I was experiencing.

Nurses went from bed to bed, doing the regular observations on every patient on the ward. This included checking blood pressure and body temperature, and other tests. They interacted with the other patients while they were doing the observations, spoke to them and reassured them. When they came to my bed, they did the tests in silence. They did not make eye contact. They did not reassure me. It was a clear representation of the way in which a patient who has attempted suicide can be treated differently. I was the only patient on the ward who was treated in this way.

I was in unimaginable pain. At the point when I most needed reassurance and comfort, it was withheld.

At one point, I desperately wanted water. I put my arm out to try to draw their attention. I could barely speak and so could only say, faintly "Water". A nurse came over to me. She said

"You've very recently had water," and walked away. I was denied water.

It felt that I was being punished, by the nurse, for causing my own internal damage.

I had effectively poisoned myself. Was it any surprise to staff that I would crave water? It is surely the body's natural response.

It was such a small request - water. It would have taken minutes for a nurse to bring it to me. It seems inhumane that this basic human need was denied.

I desperately wanted someone to hold my hand – to stay with me and hold my hand. Not a nurse or doctor – they would not have had the time – but someone. Before this overdose, I had no idea of the power of that apparently simple act.

At a time of immense pain, from which you know there is no relief, that human contact would have helped.

No one knew I was in hospital. I tried using my mobile to leave a message for one of our trustees. She had been a hospital chaplain and I instinctively called her. She later told me that the messages were incomprehensible and barely audible. The number on my mobile was withheld and she had no idea who I was, initially. However, the second inaudible message made her wonder if it was me and she phoned the hospital, discovered I was there and came in immediately. I felt so much guilt and remorse that I had attempted suicide. I felt that I had let our clients and everyone in the charity down. All I could say was sorry. I didn't have the strength to say more.

I feel it's important to make it clear that I have been permanently physically damaged by my suicide attempts (overdoses). I would not want anyone reading this to conclude that you can put large amounts of toxic substances in your body, without a high risk of permanent and debilitating internal damage.

That night a male nurse came on duty. It became clear that he was going to sit with me overnight – to watch me. One of his colleagues commented on how annoying it must be to have to sit with patients like me (patients who had attempted suicide). He said "No, I don't mind." He was the first nurse to show me any compassion or kindness during that admission. He did everything he could to make that painful night better. There are nurses who care.

In the days after a significant overdose, a person needs particular attention. You may still be experiencing the acute mental distress which led to your suicide attempt. And now you have the added effects of the internal chaos caused by the overdose, which can impact hugely upon your emotions and mental state. You are highly vulnerable in the days afterwards and may be very much at risk of a second attempt. Staff in general hospitals need to treat patients, who attempt suicide, with extreme care, and recognise the role that they can play in helping to ensure that the person does not make a second attempt, in the days after leaving hospital. Their attitude, and the way that they treat a patient, can have a significant impact on the patient's risk.

If hospital clinicians treat them differently from the other patients, then it may send a powerful message to the individual. If clinicians treat a suicidal patient less favourably, if they ignore and fail to interact with the person (as in my experience of the ward observations), deny their basic needs (water) and imply that they are an inconvenience to staff, then that is likely to reinforce the patient's belief that they don't matter, and that they have no value. They may already believe that. A depressed and suicidal person will often feel that they are worthless, and that the world would be better without them.

When the nurses carried out the observations in silence, and avoided eye contact, I felt they had made a judgment that what I had done was wrong – that I had done something reprehensible. When my request for water was denied, I felt that I was being punished for causing my own internal damage. My interpretation of their actions was that I was a bad person, who had done something wrong in attempting suicide. This increased my suicidal intent, because I wanted to obliterate this bad person. I did not want to exist, or inflict myself on the world, if I was inherently bad.

During my very first admission to a general hospital for suicidality, in 2012, I was treated in a very different way. I was treated exceptionally well, with kindness and empathy. I had been admitted purely on grounds of risk, and had not made any suicide attempts yet. As I was assessed as being at high risk of suicide, a nurse or nursing assistant sat by my bed at all times. I was being watched 24 hours a day. The care and compassion, of the nurses who were tasked with watching me, made a profound difference, on that occasion. I started to see the world as a place that I could imagine wanting to remain in. The nurses represented what is good in the world – the kindness, compassion and wish to help that represents the very best of human nature. I believe that they reconnected me with that aspect of the world.

This means that the converse can be true. Any apparently uncaring, judgmental or angry response, from a clinician or other professional that you may encounter, simply reconnects you with all the harsh unpleasant aspects of the world, which you are probably already focusing upon. I know, from personal experience, that such negative encounters have greatly increased my suicidal intent, and made an imminent attempt more likely.

These negative encounters can remind you of all the people who have previously harmed, mistreated, or inflicted pain upon you. You are focused upon this aspect of human nature.

The last person that you encounter before a suicide attempt may represent the world, at that point. They may appear to be the representative of humanity.

I wish that I could impress this upon clinicians and other professionals who may come into contact with a suicidal person. You have such a vital role, and the way that you respond to that suicidal person may make such a profound difference, in terms of the outcome, and in terms of whether they survive or not.

Recently I put up a post on the Suicide Crisis Facebook page about work that we were doing to try to highlight how some people who attempt suicide or who self-harm are not always treated with the same care and compassion as those who are admitted to hospital for other reasons. We had a meeting with general hospital management, who seemed in total denial that this could be happening to our clients, when they were admitted.

We received a comment from a member of Juliet's family, on our Facebook page, telling us that Juliet could not comment herself, since she died last year, but the family member knew that Juliet had not always been treated with compassion when she was admitted to the general hospital. Juliet had told her. It makes me so desperately sad that, while there was still a chance to help Juliet, she was treated in this way. Hospital nurses, please learn from this. Support, care and try to understand while you still can – while there is still an opportunity to help. We need to do all that we can to help each person to survive.

As well as responding with care and compassion, when a person is at risk, it is important to do all we can to try to understand the person and why they are acting in the way that they are. This is a very important part of the work that we do at Suicide Crisis.

A failure to try to understand each individual can lead to misinterpretation, and judgment, which is likely to make a person disengage - and it may mean that they don't seek help again.

I recall an example of this, from my own experience, when I was under the crisis team in the summer of 2012. I phoned them and, as there was no one available to take the call, I left a pager message for them to call me back. When a crisis team nurse returned my call an hour later, I had stopped crying and was, instead, very calm and detached. It was as if I had cut out emotionally. I feel this was probably a dissociative reaction, since I am often able to detach from my emotions, when I become particularly distressed. I told the nurse that I was okay and didn't need to talk now. His response was: "Why are you playing games with us, Joy?" The response was unhelpful, judgmental and showed a total unwillingness to try to understand what the patient is experiencing. Instead of trying to explore why my situation had changed so suddenly, he assumed that I was "playing a game". Even if I had been "playing a game" then I would expect that this is something that should be explored by the nurse to try to determine how best to help the patient. If a patient is under the care of the crisis team, then they need help and support, not judgment.

My distress an hour earlier had been acute, intense and extremely painful. This was not acknowledged or validated and I was left feeling unsupported, and chastised.

It is not difficult to see how this kind of response would make a person reluctant to phone again, if they felt distressed and at risk in the future.

There were other occasions where I felt that my mental health presentation was not understood, and I felt judged, rather than supported. This has sometimes prevented an exploration of whether my behaviour was indicative of a mental health condition.

In the summer of 2012 I displayed some impulsive, risk-taking behaviour that could have been considered "unwise". In retrospect, this is likely to have been a symptom of bipolar, which had not been considered at that point. It is common, during hypomanic or manic episodes, for a person with bipolar to engage in impulsive acts and risk-taking behaviour. I disclosed information about some risk-taking behaviour to a member of the crisis team and, instead of seeking to explore why I was engaging in this type of behaviour, which was out of character, she expressed her exasperation: "But you're a grown woman!" Her view was that my actions did not befit a person of my age and, as a grown woman, I should know better.

I learned some time afterwards that there had been a discussion later that evening amongst the crisis team about my behaviour, and I understand that some of them expressed genuine concern that I was acting in such a way. However, this was not communicated to me. I wish they had felt able to express their concern, to counteract the response of their colleague earlier that day.

In contrast, there were instances where clinicians did try to understand, and where they tried to uncover what was happening, in order that they could provide the most appropriate help. On one occasion, a mental health clinician responded in a particularly sensitive and helpful way, when I had an extreme and totally unanticipated response to a situation that arose, which was highly triggering to me.

It occurred during my first stay in psychiatric hospital, in October 2013.

I had been sitting alone in one of the communal rooms. A male nurse walked into the room, and his face immediately triggered a reaction. It looked so familiar. It took me back instantly to a place of trauma, where I felt threatened. My response was to retreat, curl up tight, and cover my face with my hands. And I wept uncontrollably, shaking with fear. He remained calm, spoke quietly and gently said: "Tell me what's happening, Joy." That phrase is so important, reflecting a wish to understand the individual's unique experience and response. If all of us, who are supporting clients at risk, work diligently to try to understand each individual under our care, then we can make such a difference. If the crisis team member, who had assumed that I was playing a game, had asked this question, then he would have perhaps been able to understand, and help.

My experiences have shown me how important it is that we work to try to understand each of our clients' unique history, responses and needs. Traumatic responses are just one example of how we may all respond differently.

On another occasion, a clinician responded in a highly effective way to my traumatic response, when I was taken ill in the countryside on a day when temperatures unexpectedly soared. An ambulance was called and the paramedics carried out some tests. I would not have anticipated that one of the actions of the paramedic would have caused such a severe reaction. Some aspects of the traumatic event may be locked inside your mind, and a seemingly innocuous incident may be triggering, and may uncover parts of the event that you could not recollect before. My physical reaction was the same as the first time – retreat, curl up small, cover my face with my hands and screw my eyes tightly closed. It is entirely instinctive. I think it must represent an attempt to protect yourself and to shut out the trauma and the person who, in that moment, you fear, because of who and what they symbolise. My reaction was far more severe this time, though, and I was distraught. The paramedic remained silent, then simply said: "You're safe now, Joy."

This simple but highly effective phrase helps to focus the patient on the present time, bringing them back from the past traumatic event that they are reliving so intensely at that moment. The danger has passed, and they are now in a safe place.

The paramedic had clearly received training in how to respond to a person who is extremely traumatised. He, and the nurse in the psychiatric hospital, both kept their distance from me and did not attempt to approach me. An untrained person may feel an instinctive reaction to come close to the patient to comfort them, perhaps even to touch them, believing that this would be reassuring. It is an entirely understandable belief, since this will often be an extremely helpful way to respond to a distressed person. However, trauma is different and, depending on the type of trauma, a human touch, when you are reliving the event, may only provoke alarm at that moment. A person approaching you may represent danger and you may struggle to distinguish between past and present or be able to recognise that the person approaching you has no connection with the traumatic event.

In both cases, the clinicians remained very focused on my individual response and they watched, waited, spoke very few words, but responded in a highly effective way.

The two examples that I have given, of positive experiences, both relate to clinicians' responses to me when I was experiencing a severe post-traumatic reaction. I find it much more difficult to find examples, from my own experience, of clinicians who worked to understand my reactions and behaviour, when suicidal. This concerns me, because I know how important it is, from my work at Suicide Crisis. Within mental health services, there seemed to be a wish to categorise and generalise, so that you conformed to a particular "type". This fails to acknowledge the complexity of the individual, or their unique reaction. If there was more focus on trying to understand each individual, it would make a difference.

If we wish to be tenacious in our attempts to help a person to survive, then it is self-evident that we should avoid giving information to a patient which assists them in ending their life.

Within the general hospital, and within psychiatric services, I have been given information about the lethality of certain suicide methods, which would directly assist me in a suicide attempt.

On one occasion I was talking to an A&E consultant about my suicide method and his response was: "That's not the most effective suicide method." I asked him to tell me what the most effective method was and, astonishingly, he told me what he thought the two most effective suicide methods were. I never expected that he would answer my question. Within a week I was at the place that he had described as being one of the two most effective ways to end my life. I didn't attempt suicide on that occasion, but he placed in my mind the idea of a method that I had not previously considered, and I was now exploring the possibility of ending my life in that way. How dangerous that information was, and how irresponsible it was to provide me with it.

On another occasion I was provided with detailed information on how to end my life. When I requested and received my own psychiatric records in 2014, I read an entry from October 2013 which gave the exact quantity of medication that a person of my weight and height would need, in order to end their life. The information came from the Cardiff Poisons Unit, so it is an extremely reliable source.

The psychiatrist, who wrote the entry in my records, had contacted the Cardiff Poisons Unit because he believed that I may have taken one of the boxes of medication, as an empty box had been discovered in my bag. He needed to find out the potential toxic effect of this quantity, and the Poisons Unit confirmed that, if I had swallowed the contents of the box, then it was a potentially fatal dose for a person of my weight and height.

Prior to reading this entry, I had believed that it would require a very large quantity of this medication in order for it to be lethal. That is what I had gleaned from the internet, from the relatively small amount of information that there is online, regarding this drug. It is not widely known as a suicide method. This entry informed me that a very small number of tablets would kill me. It is highly dangerous information for a patient to be given. I have written to my local mental health trust to advise them that they have, in effect, sent me a personalised suicide manual.

The issue is not that it is recorded in my psychiatric notes, since it was clearly important information. The issue is that information which may be harmful to a patient should be removed from a person's psychiatric records, before they receive them. A psychiatrist or psychiatrists check through a person's records, before sending them out, precisely so that this kind of detail can be removed. Two psychiatrists checked my records before they were sent out, according to the covering letter which was sent with them.

These actions serve to increase a person's risks. We need to do all that we can to minimise risks.

I have spoken before of Juliet, who died under the care of mental health services. It cannot be said that clinicians did all that they could to minimise risks and help Juliet to survive. Indeed, the inquest showed that there were significant failures.

Juliet died by suicide in the late spring – in May 2014. No client has died by suicide whilst under our care. I never want that to change. Juliet's death had such a massive impact. If she had still been under our care, it would have felt even worse.

When I found out about her death, I went into a kind of shock. That is what the psychiatrist in the mental health liaison team at the hospital wrote in her letter to my GP. I had presented at A&E, although I don't recall doing that and my discharge letter referred to the fact that my recollection of the preceding days was incomplete.

I had never felt that it was inevitable that we would lose a client. In the short time that I knew her, it was very clear that Juliet was a caring, sensitive, intuitive, perceptive woman who had so much to contribute to the world. It seemed impossible that she was not here any more.

Her inquest was in March 2015, having been adjourned from October 2014. In October it was clear that her family was going through a complaints procedure against our local mental health trust. She had been admitted to psychiatric hospital, but for only a very short time. Her husband described how he had tried desperately to have her admitted to psychiatric hospital, but no one listened. In the end he drove her to the psychiatric hospital himself and begged them to admit her. They told him that, if she had presented there alone, they would have to assess her, and staff suggested that he drive away and leave her there.

Juliet was only in hospital for a few days. She asked to leave and the hospital agreed.

At the full inquest, the coroner had called an independent psychiatrist, Dr M-W, to give evidence. His report contained a number of criticisms of our local mental health services in Gloucestershire.

His findings were as follows:-

The clinicians involved in her care had not drawn up a care plan and, when he went through her psychiatric records, he could not find a risk assessment. He emphasised that a care plan depended upon a risk assessment.

During her inpatient stays, he felt that they could have created a coordinated plan going ahead.

She had no Care Coordinator within mental health services. A Care Coordinator would have been responsible for planning and coordinating her treatment, and could have liaised with the psychiatrist at Turning Point, an independent organisation which is contracted to provide alcohol dependency services in Gloucestershire. There was no joint care plan with Turning Point and no shared understanding of what was being done.

The risks to Juliet were often minimised by mental health services, he said. Staff "took her too much on how she was on the day" and did not look at her situation in the context of what had been happening in the previous weeks and months. If she said she was okay on a particular day, they accepted that, without looking at the history of suicide attempts in the previous weeks. There was a sense of minimisation, he felt.

A community mental health team should have been involved, to give continuous care over the weeks and months, and the crisis team (Crisis Resolution and Home Treatment Team) should have set that up, and coordinated it, according to Dr M-W.

He emphasised that there should have been a clear crisis plan, which Juliet's husband should have been informed about, too.

There was little evidence of support to her husband, and no assessment of his difficulties.

The care was fragmented, he concluded.

I wrote down everything that he said. I couldn't believe it. I couldn't believe that so much had gone wrong, in terms of her care.

Three psychiatrists from our local mental health service had been required to attend the inquest and give evidence. Only two attended. Dr D is the crisis team psychiatrist and the psychiatric hospital consultant. He had been required to attend, but failed to do so, citing illness as the reason for his absence.

I can understand why he would not have wanted to attend and be questioned by the coroner. I had wanted him to be questioned, though. I feel that he should have been.

Presumably he had made decisions about her discharge. And he failed to arrange the longer term, ongoing care for Juliet that Dr M-W had said was missing, and which, he said, should have been arranged by the crisis team.

Before, and during, the inquest, no one from our mental health service would make eye contact with me, or acknowledge me, despite the fact that I was sitting in close proximity to them. They know who I am.

At the end of the inquest one of the psychiatrists, Dr C, came up to me and said: "Joy, thank you for helping that woman". Initially I didn't understand what he meant. What woman? I thought he was referring to a stranger in the waiting room outside the coroner's court. Then I realised that he meant Juliet.

His words were a strange combination of sensitivity and distance. There was a recognition, I think, on his part, that I perhaps needed to hear something comforting, at that moment. But Juliet had become 'that woman'. She no longer had a name and, it felt that she no longer had an identity to them. But this was Juliet, with all her individual and unique qualities.

I had felt a strong sense of the loss of an individual. This was a person who is irreplaceable. No one will have her unique combination of talents, her personal qualities, her individual traits.

The fact that we cared about Juliet means that her death continues to be painful for some of us, within Suicide Crisis. I would rather care, and have the resulting pain, than be so detached that the dead person becomes depersonalised.

The local press did not report all the details of Dr M-W's statement in the newspaper article. I was shocked and angry at the catalogue of failures he described, and contacted the press myself to comment. I reacted in the moment, and regret speaking to the press now. It helped no one. I am sure that this increased the wrath of our local mental health service's management and staff towards me.

I know how absolutely devastated her family are, at her loss. I spoke to some of them at her inquest and had subsequent contact with them.

I still feel intense anger at what happened, in terms of her psychiatric care.

There are other cases where I feel that more has needed to be done, in order to reduce the risks of a person dying. A striking example is Lily's story, which we took to the press in the end, in 2014, because we had tried all other routes to seek ways of ensuring that she was helped. I had contacted our mental health trust with my concerns, the CCG, her MP and had taken her case to the county suicide prevention forum.

"Lily" was the name that the local press gave to our client, in the press article. We were particularly concerned about her, because she had been self-harming to a degree that regularly put her life at risk. She was being admitted to A&E at the general hospitals several times a week, every week. She has a diagnosis of Emotionally Unstable Personality Disorder (Borderline Personality Disorder). Regular and frequent self-harm is listed in the diagnostic criteria for EUPD. The National Institute for Clinical Excellence (NICE) guidelines state that there are psychological treatments and interventions that can help reduce the incidence of self-harm amongst patients who have EUPD, including Dialectical Behaviour Therapy (DBT). However, there is no longer a DBT service in our county.

It was incomprehensible to me that Lily wasn't receiving specialist psychological therapy to help overcome her severe self-harm.

NICE recommends that counties have a specialist personality disorders unit. There is none in Gloucestershire, so I felt that she needed to be referred to a county where they do have specialist services for people with a personality disorder, and where she could access the treatment that could help her.

Lily told me that she was willing to talk to the press, anonymously, if it would raise the profile of her case and help her to access appropriate treatment. She spoke in detail about the severity of her self-harm and the fact that she had recently had a heart attack after a substantial overdose. Lily is 27.

I was interviewed by the press and stated my belief that there was a very real risk that Lily would die, if she did not receive appropriate help.

We hoped that this publicity would bring Lily the help that she needed. Our mental health service did say that they would seek a referral to a specialist hospital in London for her, after the publicity in the press. The hospital has specialist inpatient services for people with personality disorders. Patients stay there for a period of months and receive specialist therapy. Eight months after the newspaper article, she is still in Gloucestershire and nothing appears to have changed for her. She is still regularly receiving treatment in hospital and has just had an operation to remove dangerous sharp objects that she swallowed. The level and severity of her self-injury is born out of intense and overwhelming distress, and inner pain. I do not understand why she is not receiving psychological therapy to help. At a meeting that I attended, a mental health nurse stated that they acknowledge that she may kill herself through self-harm. I fail to understand why they have not ensured that she accesses appropriate treatment, which could significantly reduce the risk of this happening.

Last month I wrote to request that Lily is referred to a psychiatrist in a neighbouring county, so that he can review her treatment and make recommendations. He specialises in treating personality disorders, and has a national reputation. We are relieved to hear from Lily that this referral to the specialist psychiatrist has been agreed.

In the past year, we have had an increasing number of clients coming to us with a diagnosis of Emotionally Unstable Personality Disorder (Borderline Personality Disorder). We feel that the lack of a specialist service in this county for people with a personality disorder is the main reason behind this.

The local mental health trust's increasing antagonism towards me is perhaps explained by the adverse publicity that I had created for them. However, this negativity towards me and my charity had been long-standing, and started many months before my media interviews about client cases.

From the early days, as publicity around our Suicide Crisis Centre started (set up by a person with lived experience, who found local services had not provided what she needed), they appeared to want no official contact with us. We made attempts to contact them, but these were ignored. I was very careful to only explain in general terms, in the media and on our website, and when I gave talks, why the crisis team and mental health services, and why charities like the Samaritans, hadn't worked for me.

One of our clients said to me one day: "I defended you last week." I didn't understand, and asked her to explain. She told me that her psychologist had voiced her scepticism about our services, and our client had explained to the psychologist how helpful she had found us, and that she really respected the fact that a person, who had mental health issues and had been in crisis herself, had set up this charity. It was extremely kind of our client to do this, but it was upsetting for me to hear about this response from one of their clinicians.

Many of their clinicians seem to be unable to understand the power of lived experience, or to see it as a positive learning experience that could make a person better able to do this kind of work. It appears to be seen merely as a weakness of the charity, from their perspective.

It is interesting that we have never been asked to give a talk to our local mental health service about our work. Perhaps it is naïve of me to think that our work would be of interest to them, but you would think that it might be. It would have allowed them to have an opportunity to understand our work, rather than simply deride it, or express cynicism about it (based on assumption, rather than on any knowledge of what we do or how we work). It would give them an opportunity to understand why what we do has been effective.

However, I can perhaps understand why senior management would not have wanted that. In terms of their senior management's reaction, our mental health service seemed to see the creation of our charity as a challenge to them. I was not publicly critical of mental health services in the early days. However, they seemed to see the very existence of our charity as an implicit criticism of their services. If their services had been able to provide the right help for me, then Suicide Crisis wouldn't be needed – that seemed to be the subtext, from their perspective.

Some people outside our charity feel there is an element of fear underlying their approach to me and to our charity. I know, from reading my own psychiatric records, that they had a meeting in which they discussed whether I should be running this charity, bearing in mind my mental health issues. They questioned whether I was a suitable person to do it and whether my doing it was a risk to our clients. Frankly, they didn't know that I had bipolar at the time of this meeting in 2014, so they seemed to have very little understanding of my mental health issues anyway. And I think it is revealing that they responded in this way, by having this kind of meeting. Their conclusion was that there was no specific evidence to show that I was harmful to clients and they could find no cases of any of their patients who had been adversely affected by my support or our charity's support. Indeed we know that the opposite is true and that their patients speak so positively of our care. I wrote to our mental health trust to challenge them to find a single one of their patients (who had also used our services) who had anything negative to say about me or my charity. I also wrote: "Look at our record, and look at yours, in contrast," referring to the record of both our organisations, in terms of deaths of people under our care.

I find it so difficult to fathom why the organisation that I would have expected to understand mental illness and thus not discriminate against people who have a diagnosis seemed to be the most prejudicial – to the extent that they questioned whether I should be in the role that I am, because of my mental health issues. Is it that they need to believe that I am an 'unsuitable person' for the role? Because the alternative is perhaps too uncomfortable to contemplate – a mental health patient providing services for other mental health patients. This would turn the 'natural order' on its head. It's the psychiatrists and managers who provide mental health services – not former patients.

I think their management's increasing hostility is caused by the combination of the way in which they perceive that my role seems to challenge the normal (or accepted) order of things, and the implicit (and increasingly explicit) way that I and my charity challenge them.

Since I have been more open in raising concerns about some of their actions or services, professionals outside our charity have remarked that the trust's management seems to be showing greater hostility towards me as an individual.

In terms of our local NHS mental health services' attitude towards me and my charity, I think it involves quite a complex interplay of different factors.

The local police's attitude towards our charity, and to me, has been more straightforward. There are some police officers within our local force who are extremely empathic towards the suicidal people with whom they come into contact. They do everything that they can to help – often trying to help the individual to access appropriate care and support. There are also police officers who are not.

In 2014 I discovered that Gloucestershire Police had created an OPI, which came up on their computer screens whenever I phoned the police to request police welfare checks on our clients, or if I needed to phone them because a client was at risk from someone else. An OPI is operational information that is deemed relevant to the police. The information that came up on their screens, whenever I phoned from our charity's number was:-

"Caller Joy Hibbins   07975 ******. She claims she is part of the suicide crisis team and asks for various welfare checks. She isn't part of the team and it appears she is herself a MH patient."

It was deeply shocking to me, when I became aware that this OPI had been there for some time. I have this information in a letter from the Professional Standards department of Gloucestershire Constabulary. The OPI is quoted in the letter. It has now been amended, but its existence revealed a disturbing level of prejudice on the part of the senior officer who wrote it. Gloucestershire Police say they have been unable to identify the author of the OPI. I suspect that I will not be the only one who will feel a level of scepticism about their inability to identify the author.

The implication from the OPI is clear. It was impossible for that senior officer to imagine that a person with a mental health diagnosis could be in a responsible role within a charity. The assumption was that I must have been either delusional, or lying.

As well as being discriminatory, it put our clients at risk, because it meant that I was taken less seriously, when I phoned, by the police call handler, who saw the information on that OPI.

The police refuse to acknowledge that this is discriminatory, and I have had no apology.

A police officer once said directly to me "I don't think that you are an appropriate person to run this charity" (referring to my mental health issues).

That was an extraordinarily wounding comment, and one that I will never forget. There is definitely prejudice within the police force. However, there are large numbers of police officers in this country who genuinely care and want to help people who are either in mental health crisis or who are at risk of suicide.

The attitude of some senior police officers continued to be reflected in our local crisis care concordat. The police have a leading role in that, along with the CCG (Clinical Commissioning Group).

The CCG had already made their views clear in the early days of our charity's existence – their scepticism that a recently suicidal person, with mental health issues, could set up a Suicide Crisis Centre. I probably should not have been surprised that we were not invited to be part of the county crisis care concordat.

One day I received a text from a professional contact from another organisation: "Are you going to the launch of the crisis care concordat this afternoon?" My response was "What launch? I know nothing about it." He was shocked that I knew nothing about it, that I had not been invited, and that I had had no involvement in it, since they had been working on it for months. The county concordat is part of a national plan to ensure that organisations commit to work together to improve the system of care and support to people who are in crisis because of a mental health condition. We had been completely left out of it, despite our role in supporting people at risk of suicide, 365 days a year. Other local charities had been involved, from an early stage, but not the local charity which focuses entirely on working with people in crisis, as our name indicates.

A person who has a senior role in our county commented on the exclusion of our charity from the crisis care concordat, and our general exclusion and isolation within the county:-

"You are an authentic voice. You have a depth of knowledge and experience that most of these professionals will never have. They may have little knowledge or real understanding of issues around suicide. They are paid to be in the role that they are and, for most of them, suicide is not the main part of their role. It is not a specialism for them. Your knowledge frightens them, as does the power of what you say, because it comes from lived experience and your direct experience of working with clients."

Personally I feel that our exclusion is perhaps indicative of the fact that the commissioners were reluctant to give any acknowledgment of the existence of a crisis service that they didn't mastermind. The setting up of Suicide Crisis was a response to something that was lacking in the county. I believe that they feel that this is something that they should have perhaps identified themselves, and responded to. It is perhaps embarrassing that it took a mental health patient to set up a service that is proving to be effective and helpful to people who have struggled to find help, or who need a different type of help.

I have found that reasoning very difficult to hold onto, though. The accumulative effect (of the many times that I have been excluded) has impacted severely upon me. It continues to affect me.

This isolation, not just of our charity, but particularly of me, as an individual, had a hugely detrimental effect. There had been so many incidences of prejudice and exclusion. I felt that I was the reason behind the exclusion, since I have a mental health diagnosis – indeed, more than one mental health diagnosis.

I felt that I was perceived as tainted in some way, as if I was damaged by my diagnoses. It felt that this was the reason behind the continual rejection of our charity. If I was not running it, it would be accepted.

It is well documented that isolating a person can increase the risk of suicide, and I was clearly being ostracised. I felt that I was a burden to my charity and the barrier to its acceptance in the county. Without me, it would thrive. I felt that I was nothing – that I was not good enough. Friends pointed to the success of the charity, and the excellent feedback of our clients. I couldn't hear it. The isolation of our charity and of me, along with the comments that I have already documented, made by people within the powerful organisations – all of this seemed to gradually accumulate and overpower me.

These were triggers that sent me into a depressive low, and into a suicidal place. By admitting this, I am probably reinforcing what they might wish to promote – that I am 'mentally fragile'. I wonder how they would respond themselves, if they had experienced the level of exclusion that I have experienced. Yes, I have bipolar disorder and that means that I will repeatedly experience depressive episodes. And, if you have bipolar, there may be triggers to such episodes. I now know that continual rejection and isolation of our charity can be a trigger. It has been a learning experience and, as a result, I am careful about the contact that I have with these powerful individuals and organisations now.

It is such a sad irony that the actions of those leading the crisis care concordat and the county suicide prevention forum, whose task is to reduce the number of suicides and provide appropriate help in crisis situations, impacted upon me so much that I wanted to end my life.

Some of the members of the county suicide prevention forum gradually felt that Suicide Crisis should be part of the forum. My understanding is that pressure was exerted upon Public Health officials, who lead it, and we were invited to join in 2014. I attended two meetings and, at the second, I felt that the attitude of the Public Health officials, who led the forum, had not changed. One of the members pointed out that the contact details of Suicide Crisis were not in a crucial county document on suicide, which Public Health had created. We were still being sidelined and excluded, despite being at meetings. There were other examples of this exclusion, at the meeting.

Even after the forum member pointed out this omission, Suicide Crisis was not included in the document.

As I am aware that an accumulation of these types of incidents can trigger a depressive episode, I decided not to attend further meetings. Suicide Crisis left the county suicide prevention forum.

Outside the county, the response to our charity, and to me, has been very different. Our charity has been welcomed and appreciated.

I felt honoured to be invited to meetings of the All Party Parliamentary Group on Suicide and Self-Harm, and to have the opportunity to contribute to discussions at these meetings.

As I travelled up on the train to my first meeting, I remember feeling that I was sure that I would not have the courage to speak at that meeting, but that I would be happy to listen. I also thought of how interested and excited my parents would have been to know that I was travelling to a meeting in Parliament. My parents first met at a Labour Party meeting. They were passionate and idealistic and hoped to change things for the better, via political means. Everything seemed possible to them. They would have loved to hear about the politicians that I had met and the subjects that we discussed.

In the event, the subject matter of that first meeting was so important to me that I did speak, and in some detail.

At my second meeting, I was equally nervous. Once again, however, I felt moved to speak. All went well initially, until I had a sudden realisation: "I'm a mental health patient from Gloucestershire, speaking in Parliament before Norman Lamb, and other extremely important ministers and eminent professors." And I totally froze at the sudden realisation of where I was. Moments passed and people met my gaze. And then my eyes focused on Madeleine Moon, who was chairing the meeting. She smiled at me. That gave me the reassurance that I needed to continue. Both Madeleine Moon and Norman Lamb were very kind to me at that meeting.

I also had a separate meeting with Norman Lamb and his personal assistant on another day and I am extremely grateful for the interest that he showed in Suicide Crisis. Norman suggested that I make contact with Louis Appleby, the Government's adviser on suicide, and also with a psychiatrist who was tasked with running the South West Zero Suicide Initiative, one of three pilot schemes for the Government's Zero Suicide initiative.

My subsequent meeting with Louis Appleby was productive and interesting. I was surprised (and impressed) by the honesty with which he spoke, and his willingness to stray into difficult areas of conversation, on issues related to suicide and mental health provision in this country.

The psychiatrist, who was leading the South West Zero Suicide Initiative, had already been in contact with our charity, to suggest that we gave a presentation to their steering committee. We gave a presentation to both their steering group and reference group, and they described our work as "extraordinary" and "inspirational".

"Inspirational" was the word that kept being repeated, and it was such a shock to me to have such a positive reaction, when I was so used to being excluded by the people of influence in my own county.

My friend and colleague, V, accompanied me at that presentation. V provides clinical supervision to some of our team members, and advises us on various matters relating to our work. She is a psychiatric nurse, nurse manager and has had a lead position in a psychological therapies service.

We were at university together but lost touch in our twenties. V found me again in 2012, via Facebook. It was strange and fortuitous timing that she contacted me during a period when her professional background would have a particular significance. She was an ideal person to approach in 2013, when we started offering services, and she readily agreed to do what she could to help our charity.

I think it must be extremely difficult for my friends to see the contrast between the person that I was at university, and the person that I am now. At university I had not been touched by mental illness, or suicidal thoughts or intent. I still remember clearly the reference that one of my tutors wrote for me at the end of my university degree: "She provided a strong and stable presence in a somewhat nervous year." I wonder how he would react, if he knew my recent history. I also remember that he wrote that my "gentle appearance and manner" masked an inner strength. If you are gentle in your approach, people do not immediately see strength. It is very easy to be underestimated and overlooked, if you are gentle. I have found gentleness to be such a helpful quality, when supporting people who are extremely traumatised. It is not a quality that is often highlighted, appreciated or prized, in today's world.

I remember talking to a professional contact about gentleness, and I spoke about the fact that I value it so much in members of our team. She commented that gentleness was okay, "as long as it doesn't equate to 'ineffective'". It isn't ineffective. It can be hugely powerful, in the same way that kindness can be immensely powerful.

The recognition of our work by influential people outside our county has been so appreciated. But it is the feedback from our clients that matters to us. Indeed, that is ultimately all that matters – their experience and the fact that they feel helped. We are constantly told that clients don't feel that they could have survived, without our charity. This charity works because of a unique combination of factors, not least the connection that we have with our clients and the relationship with a person or people who they trust, who cares about them and their survival, who seeks to understand, in an organisation where the support is tailored to their individual needs as much as possible. Our exceptional team is at the heart of this. We have chosen highly skilled individuals, who are also particularly caring, insightful and giving people- each of them unique, but all of them giving selflessly of their time.

There are times when clients are at high risk, and members of our team have spent many hours past their regular work commitment, in order to help ensure that a client remains safe. It's because we care and, as said before, we are tenacious in the way that we help clients to survive. I am so indebted to our team for their commitment.

It is hugely important that our clients know that we care about them and about their survival. It has sometimes felt to me, from my experiences, that there may be a fear, on the part of mental health clinicians, of showing that they care about their patients. It is as if they fear that some barrier will be crossed, that will lead to confusion and misunderstanding of the boundaries of the professional relationship. It doesn't, in our experience. It is totally possible to have a professional relationship, where you care.

I recall one occasion when I was under the NHS crisis team, and one of their nurses was talking to me on the phone. She was concerned about my imminent risk. "I'm not afraid to say that I care," she said. It was a revealing comment, I felt. The implication was that her colleagues were afraid to show that they cared.

We rarely need to say that we care. Clients know that we do, and they tell us this.

It means that our work is painful, at times, because we fear that we may lose a client. The silent waiting for news of a client, who is at a location of high risk, can be extremely difficult. The same applies when a client is missing, and suicidal. And if a client is in hospital after a suicide attempt, there may be many hours of waiting for news of whether they will survive.

We work in situations of imminent risk. A new client may contact us, at the point of suicide, sometimes from the location where their plan could be carried out immediately and quickly.

This was the case with one young woman who contacted us while she was on the way to the place where she intended to end her life. It became clear that she was in Gloucester, but in this city there is more than one of the type of location to which she was referring. I don't know Gloucester very well. I was born there and lived there as a young child, and consider my roots to be in Gloucester, but I don't know it geographically in terms of landmarks and streets. She told us broadly which part of the city she was in, but didn't indicate her precise location or her intended destination.

I contacted the police and could give the general district where she was, but this covered a wide area. I remained on the phone to the woman at risk, but went to speak to Justin, the psychological therapist who runs our PTSD group, as they were coming to the end of their meeting. I asked him if he knew Gloucester. Like me, he didn't know it well and lived in Cheltenham. However, Natalie, who attends the PTSD group, overheard me and told us that she lived there and was familiar with the area that I was asking about.

This created the unprecedented situation of another client assisting us in trying to identify where the woman at risk was heading. We knew Natalie well. She was a caring, calm, practical, level-headed woman, who was not suicidal or at risk herself, and so I explained the situation to her and the type of place the woman was trying to access. Natalie explained that there were two similar places near the area where the woman was.

By now the police had asked Justin to stay on another phone to them so that he could pass on information to the police from me, as I remained on the phone to the woman.

It is an intensely pressurised situation when you are on the phone to a person that you don't know, who is walking to the place where she intends to kill herself. My focus was on engaging her, building a connection with her, ensuring that she stayed with me all the time and didn't end the call. If it is a client that we have got to know and understand, who is at imminent risk, then we already have a connection, and it is this prior connection and understanding of our client's situation that is so helpful at this time. They know and trust us, and already have a relationship with our team. In a situation where a new client contacts us in such a high risk situation, we must work very quickly to build rapport and trust.

Natalie played a key role in helping us to give vital information to the police. The three of us were now working together (Justin, Natalie and I). We needed Natalie's geographical knowledge.

The police started to give Justin instructions to pass onto me. They wanted me to ask her questions about her location. I wanted to do this in a way that didn't alarm her or tell her that we were seeking to send help to her because she was still adamant that she did not want this to happen. It was a fragile situation and I did not want to cause her to end the call. So I asked her to describe what was happening around her and what she could see. From her brief description, it sounded like an industrial park. I repeated out loud the description she gave me and Natalie identified immediately where she was, and Justin passed this onto the police.

Natalie had felt that our new client was heading to one of two possible destinations. The police had not located her and so I was continuing to try to get a geographical sense of where she was, without her becoming alarmed that services were suddenly going to descend upon her. I have no idea how long this continued. I am unable to put a time frame upon it, as I was so completely absorbed in the situation, as it was unfolding.

I remember the point where I could tell that her pace was quickening. I could hear it in her breathing and I knew that she must be close to her destination. She must be able to see it now, I thought, and she is walking with more determination because it is in her sight. There is so much that goes through your head at that point. It is difficult to describe the emotions that you feel in those seconds, when you know that a person may be moments away from ending their life and you personally are nowhere near them. And at the same time you are thinking "Where are the police?" "Where are they?"

Then I heard Justin say: "The police are with her."

It is such an immense sense of relief, when you know that a person is safe.

Natalie played a key role that night. Her knowledge of Gloucester was invaluable. I do not know whether we would have been able to help the police to locate her quickly enough, without Natalie's involvement.

In most cases of clients at high risk, we are the ones going out to them. When a person calls us for the first time, and it is clear that they are at imminent risk, two of us go out, after assessing the risks by talking to the person on the phone first. However, I recall an instance when only I was available.

It was a Saturday night and I received a call from a woman who was clearly extremely distressed, and under the influence of alcohol. She described her plan to end her life that night. She had recently been in the psychiatric hospital and wanted to return there.

I talked to her about going to A&E at the general hospital because I felt it was the right place to go initially. She had used alcohol and I knew that this meant that psychiatric staff wouldn't do an assessment until the effects of alcohol had diminished. And I knew that she could gain admission to the psych hospital via the general hospital and explained this to her. But she was fearful of going there.

I knew that I needed to go out to her, but my regular 'partner' (my professional partner who accompanied me on night emergency work) was on a night out in Birmingham.

Fortunately another colleague, who also sometimes did outreach work with me, was able to take me out to the woman at risk, but he had already told me that he would have to leave me there as he had other commitments. The woman's husband had now also phoned saying that he felt that the situation was deteriorating. He felt that we could encourage her to come to the general hospital if I went out there. I assured him that I was on my way.

I arrived at their home and went inside. She was extremely distressed and I spoke to her for some time. We spoke about going to the general hospital and she said: "If I go, will you stay with me at the hospital?" I reassured her that I would.

We spent many hours in A&E waiting that night – all three of us – and we were able to talk at length. She spoke in detail about the reasons why she had wanted to end her life that night.

I remember, though, that she totally unsettled me, quite late into the night, by her reaction to the fact that I was myself a survivor of suicidal crisis. Another organisation had signposted her to us, she said, but it was clear that the organisation had misunderstood how our charity works. She had been told that we were an organisation of survivors whose role was to demonstrate that a person 'can come out the other side'. Apparently our role was to show, by example, that a person could come through a suicidal crisis.

That's a misunderstanding, by the referring professional, of our charity. Our team is not made up of survivors of suicidal crisis and one cannot assume that it would necessarily always make a person feel less suicidal if they knew that another person had come through a crisis. I personally found it no help, when I was absolutely at the point of wanting to die, to be told that other people had survived suicidal crises. I could not relate to that, nor relate it to my own situation.

She gazed at me very intently and said two words: "You know." It was unnerving. "You know, don't you? I can see it in your eyes."

It was as if she could see into my soul, and could observe what I had experienced.

At around 4am she was admitted to a ward and I knew that she would be safer and more comfortable there. It is so easy to walk out of A&E when you are a suicide risk. The staff don't necessarily have time to monitor you and it can be a busy, noisy, distressing environment, even when you are on a bed in one of the cubicles, as our client was. It can be difficult to stay in that environment, when you are already distressed. The woman at risk had expressed a wish to leave several times while we were in A&E, and that's why I felt it important to stay with her.

She visibly relaxed when she was in the ward and I knew that I could leave now. As I told her I was leaving, she took my hand and asked me to promise to return the next day, and I reassured her that we would come back the next day on the ward to see her. This initial connection and rapport is so important. If a person can connect with us, we can be part of their continuing sense of connection to the world, at a time when a larger part of them is trying so hard to disconnect from it, and leave it.

A smaller number of us do this kind of night work. However, all of my colleagues have spent many hours, when they have needed to, with a client who is at imminent risk during our core hours which are up until 10pm. They do this because they care and want to do everything that they can to help our clients to survive.

The two examples, that I have cited, give an idea of how we might respond to an initial call from a person who is at imminent risk of suicide, when they are unable to come to our crisis centre. However, it is, of course, sometimes the case that a client, who we have already been supporting for a while, will have a triggering incident that suddenly increases his or her risk. I recall going out, at very short notice, to the home of a client who we had been supporting at our Trauma Centre, because it was clear that he was at risk that night. He was under the care of a mental health team, as well as being supported by us. Early on that evening, he suddenly became angry, exclaiming that "None of you professionals know what it is really like to have PTSD." I rarely reveal personal information, or information about my own history to clients, but I felt it was appropriate, in this situation, to tell him that I had PTSD. I think he had felt so isolated with his condition, had struggled to understand it (as we all do, initially), felt that he could never recover and function as he used to. I said nothing other than the fact that I had PTSD and answered one other question from him about it, but I felt that it was a time when it could help for him to know this. We talked for an extended period of time until I felt it was safe to leave, and we arranged that I would call at fixed points later that night, to ensure that he was continuing to feel safe.

The work that we do relating to imminent risk often occurs at night or in the early hours of the morning, when a known client contacts us. This is usually via our emergency nightline, which is available to a small number of our clients who are not using any other services and who have made it clear that they would not call anyone else in the night, if they were at imminent risk.

As I am on call at night several nights a week, I am able to sleep because I know that the phone is very loud and will wake me within seconds. Clients often comment, after the crisis is over, that they were surprised that it was only seconds before the phone was answered. I'm a light sleeper, which is useful in these circumstances.

The name of the caller immediately comes up on the screen when a client calls. We are aware of the clients who are particularly high risk during a certain time period, so the name of the client is not usually a total surprise, but occasionally it is, because something has triggered a dramatic change in the circumstances of a client who had been recovering – or because they are at risk from someone else. A number of our clients have experienced domestic violence from a partner. There are also some clients who are at risk of violence from criminal gangs. A violent or potentially violent incident could happen at any time of the day or night. Some of our clients have had their lives threatened, and live in fear every night of their lives. It is not always one of our clients who has been involved in criminal activity, but a member of their family, and our client has become a target as a result of their connection to the family member.

I have to awaken very rapidly. And I have to be able to function well and think very clearly within seconds of awakening. These are exceptionally difficult calls to take, because this is a person that we know, who may be at the point of taking their own life. It is someone with whom we have a connection, and who we care about.

An unexpected call came one night from a client who had been at high risk of suicide a few weeks earlier. Things had been improving for him. He was a client who was adamant that he would not seek other help or support. He feared that it would impact upon his job and future prospects if there was a record at his GP surgery that he had been suicidal. This meant that he would also not access mental health services.

He had concerned us very much because he had access to a suicide method that was no longer readily available, which was very reliable and which would lead to his death. He had shown strong intent a few weeks before this night.

He was distraught when he called. He was out in the countryside in driving rain. He had walked for miles and was now walking through fields. There was a real sense of immediate danger. The connection that we already had was vital that night. Indeed, he told me later that he felt he could not end his life without speaking to us first. We had done so much for him, he said, and had tried so hard to help. He knew that we genuinely cared.

We talked, and I encouraged him to walk back to the road, while I remained with him on the phone. We continued to talk for about an hour and I felt that the imminent risk had reduced. He told me that he felt safe to walk home now and that he would call me in about an hour's time, when he arrived home. Just over an hour later he called and told me he was wrapped in a duvet with a hot drink, and we talked some more until he started to feel tired, and felt that he would be able to rest now.

When a client is away from home, it is always very unpredictable, and much more difficult to get help for them, if they do attempt suicide. If a client is distressed and has left home, they may no longer be sure of their location – or they may withhold that information. I recall a client who was in contact with me by phone for several hours one day. She was no longer in Gloucestershire. She told me that she was in South Wales but would not give me any further information about her location.

She informed me that she had taken an overdose of tablets. I knew that, with this particular medication, there was an eight hour period in which an antidote could be administered. After eight hours have passed, it may be too late for medical staff to save the life of that person. Although she remained in contact with me for the seven hours after taking the overdose, she would not tell me where she was. It is always extremely distressing to hear when a client has taken this particular overdose. If it doesn't kill them, it will, in a large dose, cause massive permanent internal damage.

We had reached the point where there was only an hour to go before the eight hour period was over. I spoke to her, tried to persuade her to give me her location. She wouldn't give it. I could feel tears rolling down my cheeks as I realised that our client, who we knew well, and who we cared about, may now die. Time was running out. It had nearly run out because it would take time to get an ambulance to her, and transport her to a hospital. She didn't appear to hear the emotion in my voice as I continued to speak to her.

Forty minutes before the deadline was up, she agreed to be helped. She was admitted to hospital, received medical care, and recovered.

It is usually the case that our clients find us. They hear about us or are referred to us or find us on the internet, or see something in the press about us. However, occasionally we find them.

One night I was leaving the general hospital after visiting the out of hours GP surgery. As I walked out of the building, I became aware of a man slumped against the wall of the hospital, outside Accident and Emergency. I went over to him just to check that he was okay. He explained that he had been in A&E. He had been admitted after falling in the town centre. An ambulance had been called which took him to hospital. He told me that he had found it difficult in A&E and that is why he had come outside. He didn't feel that he had been treated with respect by some of the staff and he felt that this was because he had drunk a large amount of alcohol.

A security guard came out, as we were talking, and told him that if he wasn't going to come into A&E then he should leave the hospital grounds. This concerned me, because the man was under the influence of alcohol, was having difficulty standing, and had suffered a fall which meant ambulance staff felt that he needed to be taken to A&E.

The man asked the security guard whether he had ever served in the armed forces in Afghanistan or Iraq. He explained that, if he had, he might understand why he was in the situation that he was now. The security guard told him that he hadn't and made a dismissive remark that I felt was unhelpful and inappropriate. I could no longer keep silent at this point and told the guard that I felt this was unhelpful and I did not feel the man was well enough to leave the premises. The guard then focused on me and questioned what I was doing in the hospital grounds and asked me to leave. The man, with whom I had been talking, politely but firmly told the guard not to speak to me in that way – that I was a lady and was trying to help him. I found the conduct of the security guard extraordinary.

The man and I both remained where we were. The security guard seemed unsure what to do and so went back inside the hospital. This gave us the opportunity to talk some more and the man told me how he was haunted by nightmares and images of what he had experienced during the wars he had fought in. He drank to try to block out these images and prevent him from thinking about what he had witnessed.

It sounded as if he was describing very clear symptoms of PTSD. I'm not a clinician but it was enough to make me feel it was a possibility.

He told me that he lived in one of the hostels for men who are homeless. At this point an empathic nurse came out and encouraged him to come back into the hospital so that they could assess him properly, and so I left, but I continued to think about what he had revealed to me.

I had had some contact with the hostel where the man had told me he lived, and so I went there the next day. The man had given me his first name and so I wrote a letter to him which I took in to the hostel. Staff told me that they would give it to him.

A couple of days later I heard back from the man. He had asked hostel staff how he could contact me and they gave him the charity's mobile number. In my letter I had thanked him for the way in which he had spoken to the security guard when he had told me to leave the hospital grounds. He had been polite but very firm and very clear in his message to the security guard. The security guard had said things that were quite inflammatory, but the man had remained calm and had continued to put his point across, trying to explain and make the security guard understand. To be able to do that, when you are in a highly vulnerable situation, was impressive. That was the main focus of my letter. I let him know about our trauma services but just very briefly. He had told me that people who use alcohol are often treated like 'scum' by professionals. I had felt there were parallels between the way people who use alcohol may be responded to, and the way people who are suicidal (or who have attempted suicide) are sometimes responded to, by professionals. We may both evoke anger, derision and irritation in them. I did not express any of this to the man, as my own experience would not be relevant or helpful.

His reply was that he was not used to being thanked – or having anyone say positive things about him. Having spent two and a half years under mental health services, where I was often told what I was doing wrong, and where almost nothing positive was said about me during the whole of that time, I can relate to what he was saying. Many of us who are accessing services may already feel that we are nothing. We don't need services to reinforce that belief. I wonder why statutory services do not do more to seek to challenge that belief and help us to see our value and our individual strengths and personal qualities.

When I was under mental health teams, I felt that mental health clinicians did not acknowledge positive qualities in me, whilst frequently pointing out negative aspects, and telling me how I was failing. For this reason, I know how important it is that we recognise and appreciate the individual qualities of our clients at our Suicide Crisis Centre, and ensure that they know that we see these positive qualities, since they may no longer be able to see them, particularly if they are depressed.

Our work can take us to many different locations. However, most of our clients come in to see us at our Suicide Crisis Centre. We can usually arrange to see people at very short notice. A distressed client, who is at risk, will often come in straight away. They can then come in to see us as often as they like and this may be every day for a period of time, until they feel safer.

The work can be harrowing and I recall, in particular, a woman who came to us a few weeks ago, who had been raped. She came in to see us within a couple of hours of her first phone call. She spoke in detail about what had happened to her during the assault, which happened a few weeks earlier. This is always extraordinarily difficult to hear. You cannot help but be affected personally by hearing the person's account of events, and witnessing their distress. She had reached the decision that she wanted to go to the police to report the crime, and we spoke about how we could support her through this.

It is the cases of sexual assault that I find most difficult. It is particularly upsetting to hear about cases where a client has attempted to bring charges against the person who assaulted them, but has been unsuccessful. The impact upon the victim (of not being able to hold the person to account for what they have done) can be catastrophic.

One of the first clients who came to us when our Suicide Crisis Centre opened in the autumn of 2013 was a woman who had been the victim of domestic violence.

She told us about her two teenage daughters. They had both been sexually assaulted in childhood by her ex-partner. They had recently told their mum about the assaults and she had supported them while they made statements to the police about what had happened.

The police reached a decision that there was not enough evidence to take the case forward. My understanding, from our client, was that her daughters "had not been able to give enough detail" about the assaults and had not been able to give enough information about when the incidents happened.

I read the police reports of the interviews and it was clear that one of the girls, in particular, had given a very detailed account of the sexual assaults. It was extremely upsetting to read. I cannot imagine what greater "detail" the police would have required in order to pursue the case. And in terms of dates, I wonder why there is an expectation that a person would necessarily be able to set the historic abuse in a precise time frame. The attacks had happened when they were of primary school age. Unless they can relate the assaults to particular events that were happening at the time, which would indicate the month and year that they happened, then it may be difficult to be precise. If an individual has experienced shock, terror and profound emotional turmoil, then this may make it difficult to recall exactly when the incidents happened. There are many reasons why a person may not recollect exact dates.

Our client brought both of her daughters in subsequently so that we could arrange support for them. Rape Crisis agreed that one of their counsellors would come into our Crisis Centre every week to support the elder daughter. The younger daughter did not want to seek specialist support yet, but we arranged ongoing support which did not relate specifically to the assaults. When the younger daughter first came in to see us, so that we could assess what kind of support would be most helpful, she spoke to us about the sexual assaults – not the intricate detail of what happened, but the fact that the assaults had occurred and the impact upon her. I had no doubt that she had been sexually assaulted. She was so totally credible, both in terms of what she described and the effect upon her of speaking about it. It is very difficult to accept that she has not been able to bring her attacker to justice.

Another of our clients had been the victim of historic sexual abuse and was going through the legal system to bring criminal charges. In her case, the police had told her that it would be going to court, but several months into the investigation this changed, and she told us that the police had informed her that they had not been able to accumulate enough evidence from witnesses in order to proceed. She was devastated. She called us on the emergency line on the night that the police told her this. She was distraught, and wanted to end her life. Her lawyer had told her that he felt that she should now bring a civil case against her attackers, but she told us that she had no fight left in her to do so. We supported her through that night, and, after taking a period of time to recover, she made a decision to pursue a civil case against those responsible for the crimes against her.

As we run a Trauma Centre, as well as a Suicide Crisis Centre, we see a high proportion of clients who have been the victim of domestic violence. Sometimes we become involved in a situation where there is an immediate risk of harm to our client. One young woman had been supported at our centre, because she had experienced domestic violence from a previous partner and this had impacted severely upon her. She described her current partner as very controlling, and extremely possessive, which made her concerned. One afternoon I received a single text from her. The first line of the text was: "I need help. I can't call the police. I can't ring them." The text alerted me to the fact that her partner was "getting nasty". "I feel like he's gonna kick off."

I texted back that I was calling 999 and asked if she could get out of the house. It was clear that she couldn't. We were texting each other within seconds. Then three minutes later I received one which read: "He's attacked me." "Hurry pls." I contacted 999 again to urge them to get there quickly. Another text came from our client: "They need to hurry." I asked if she could get to a safe room: "No". And two minutes later: "They're not here" (meaning the police). At this point the texts stopped. I continued to text her but received no replies. After my second 999 call the police had remained on the phone to me. I remember saying to them "She's not answering." There was just silence.

Those silent moments, waiting, were horrendous. I feared that she might be dead.

Ten minutes passed before the police were able to confirm to me that they were on the scene and that our client was injured, but alive.

Her partner was arrested and charged.

Her case highlights coercive control, in a relationship, and how that can create particular risks. Coercive control may mean that there are no acts of violence – until finally a violent attack occurs which may be so extreme that it leads to the death of the victim. New laws are now being created which give police powers to intervene where there is evidence of coercive control (even if there is no violence) within a relationship. It is so important that we all become more aware of the risks that surround this form of control.

The relationship has now ended and our client is slowly rebuilding her life.

We have another client who has been the victim of severe and life-threatening violence from her ex-partner. He has made direct threats against her life and the police are very aware of the risk to her, if he finds her. Although my colleague is her main support, I have also supported her and I will never forget the details of the domestic violence that she described, since it is so extreme. She has received ongoing support at our Crisis Centre. There are times when she has been at high risk of suicide.

A significant number of our clients who have experienced an extremely traumatic event or events use alcohol or substances in an attempt to block out the painful memories. This is particularly true of clients who have Post-Traumatic Stress Disorder. Alcohol is sometimes used to try to block out the intrusive thoughts, and the distressing images that they experience as flashbacks. This was the case with the man who was slumped outside the general hospital, who had been in the army. It is also the case for a number of our other clients.

We remember, in particular, our client who died of the effects of alcohol. She died of pancreatitis.

She first came to us in the summer of 2013. She had heard about our PTSD group and attended the very first meeting.

At the second meeting, she spoke about how she felt about the group. She told us that she had attended a number of groups over the years, but it was the first time that she had attended a group where she felt really accepted. She described having felt, for years, that she was an "ugly duckling", but it was as if the other group members had said "It's okay. You're a swan. Come and join us." She felt valued and accepted, and she was amongst people who could understand and relate to the post-traumatic world that she inhabited.

In those early days of attending the group, she was not drinking. She had been using alcohol, but she described how she felt that she was recovering. She was being supported by alcohol services and mental health services.

I recall the day that things changed for her. She attended a PTSD group meeting and it was clear that she was heavily under the influence of alcohol. She told us that she had been to an alcohol support group meeting earlier that day (within statutory services) and she had been extremely distressed by listening to another member of the alcohol support group. She had found it quite traumatic and had been drinking since the meeting, as it had destabilised her so much.

Her situation deteriorated rapidly after that. She began to drink large quantities of alcohol every day. Her post-traumatic symptoms were worsening and that was why she was using alcohol. In particular, she told us, she drank heavily at night because of the horrific "night terrors" that she experienced. She would awake to find herself out of bed, totally disorientated.

I repeatedly contacted local mental health services to say that she was seeking a formal assessment for PTSD. My understanding was that one of their psychologists had felt that she had PTSD but she had not had a psychiatrist's opinion, and therefore there was no formal record of the diagnosis.

We provided one to one support at our Crisis Centre initially, but she started to miss appointments, and so I and a colleague arranged home visits.

She desperately wanted to be able to access residential rehab where she would not just be treated for her alcohol dependency, but also for the post-traumatic symptoms that she was trying to mask by using alcohol.

However, it was clear that she was not going to be able to access any kind of residential rehab. She was told that she needed to engage with statutory services in the community first. She needed to attend her outpatient appointments for alcohol dependency to provide evidence to them that she was "engaging with them, and making progress".

Her alcohol intake at this point was so high that she was unable to leave the home, though. She had reached a point where she was so unwell that she couldn't 'make progress' on her own, alone, at home. Surely this is the point where a person needs to be able to receive intensive support in a residential setting. The person is in crisis and there should be crisis intervention for people who are so alcohol dependent that they are no longer able to function.

Local alcohol services told me that they would never be able to 'present a case' to the board for her accessing residential rehab, while she was not attending appointments in the community. I emailed them and asked: "Can I go and stand before the board? I'll put a case for her."

Her GP, social services and indeed all services told me that it was "her choice" to continue to drink. They all used that phrase. I pointed out that she had been prescribed anti-depressants, so she was clearly clinically depressed, and she was drinking to try to block out harrowing and distressing post-traumatic symptoms. I felt that I was a lone voice, both at the meetings I attended with those agencies about our client, and in the email and other communications that I had with them.

They told me that she needed to "show motivation" to give up drinking. My reply was that a lack of motivation was often an inherent part of clinical depression. It was as if they were saying: "Shake off your depression and then we'll help you." How was that ever going to happen?

Mental health services stopped supporting her. It appeared to happen very abruptly. She was told that their support was ending and they would start supporting her again when she had demonstrated that she had been free of alcohol for a month. They told me that they felt this would be an "incentive" for her to reduce her alcohol intake. She was devastated. She told me that she felt abandoned by them. The consequence, for her, was that she felt the situation was hopeless and she drank even more.

Many months before her death, a meeting was arranged by social services, which involved the different agencies supporting her. Towards the end of the meeting I was told that it was likely that Suicide Crisis would be, ultimately, the only organisation which continued to support her. "I know that must be very difficult for you to hear," the person leading the meeting told me.

In the months before she died, she was admitted to hospital multiple times as a result of accidents and falls. I recall going out to her home with a colleague and finding her bruised, bleeding and confused. We called an ambulance and she was admitted to hospital. Every time she was admitted to hospital, I flagged this up with the other agencies, including social services. I thought that surely someone would intervene to provide significant help in this ongoing crisis situation.

Ten days before she died, I spoke to our client on the phone: "Joy, I'm fading fast," she said. I emailed all the services involved in her care and told them very clearly that she would die – and soon – if something wasn't done urgently. Ten days later she was dead.

I feel that her death was entirely preventable. It is incomprehensible to me that there is not intensive, residential treatment for people who, as in the case of our client, are unable to stop drinking without significant support, because they have severe mental health issues. I feel that I watched her slowly die, feeling utterly helpless, since we could not provide treatment for her mental health or alcohol issues.

If she had received this kind of residential help months earlier, then could her death have been prevented? I have no medical knowledge but it seems to me that her body would have been saved from many more months of internal damage, and her death might not have occurred.

I attended her funeral and heard someone say: "There are some people who are beyond help." I disagree. She was not "beyond help". She was just unable to access the right kind of help.

None of us is "beyond help". We have simply not been offered the type of help that would have made a difference for us.

Sometimes clients come to us who have been categorised by mental health services as "difficult to engage". However, they engage immediately with us, demonstrating perhaps that the previous approach of the other service may simply have not been right for them. We are all individuals, with different needs.

I encountered a psychiatrist within our local mental health service who recognised this. He was a locum clinician, and he was only in post for a few months, before he was offered a permanent position in another part of the country.

He realised, from reading my psychiatric records, that I had not appeared to have found mental health services helpful. So he told me that he was going to try a different approach.

"I'm just going to work with the person I have in front of me," he said.

Instead of trying to categorise or label me, he saw me as an individual and worked with that individual.

He talked to me as if I were an equal. This was very different from the approach that I had encountered with previous psychiatrists. He didn't talk to me as though he was in a position of power, or as though he was all-knowing and I should just accept everything he said because he was the "expert".

He tried to get to know me and understand what kind of person I was.

I had a sense of being heard, which I had not felt until then.

Significantly, he pointed out positive qualities in me. This was not something that I had experienced from other mental health clinicians.

He was supportive of the work that I was doing within Suicide Crisis. This was, again, such a different approach from the rest of the clinicians and staff in our local mental health service.

He arranged to see me every week and I engaged well with him.

For a short period of time, I had a type of mental health care that worked for me. The psychiatrist demonstrated that it is not that a patient is "difficult to engage". If we provide something that meets their individual needs, then the patient will engage.

A patient may also disengage from mental health services because they have not been correctly diagnosed. If they don't have the correct diagnosis then they are unlikely to get the right treatment. I had to fight very hard to get a diagnosis of PTSD.

Bipolar was obviously completely missed by my own mental health services.

We are frequently contacted by individuals who are concerned about the suicide risk of a family member or friend. On some occasions, they have told us that they feel that their relative or friend is showing symptoms of a particular mental health condition, but find that the professionals do not listen when they point this out. They fear that the lack of correct diagnosis may mean that the person concerned is not receiving the right treatment. When I was assessed in Oxford, the psychiatrists specifically wanted to speak to a family member or close friend of mine, because clinicians recognised that it is often close relatives who will have noticed the bipolar highs and lows, rather than the patient. They were seen to have a significant role in providing information to the psychiatrist, which would help them to diagnose. I wish that all psychiatrists would value the information provided by relatives and friends.

They provide a unique insight, since they may be with the person every day. They can observe ongoing patterns of behaviour, and changes in behaviour, and they have a detailed knowledge and understanding of the person which is very different from that of a psychiatrist.

In my case, it was indeed a friend who first suggested to me that I may have bipolar. He had been able to observe that I went from a deep depression to a significant high, within the space of a few days. Bipolar would never have occurred to me, until he mentioned it. It was his comment that led me to approach GPs, who referred me for psychiatric assessment in Oxford.

It is so important that we recognise and value the input of friends, relatives and carers.

Caring for a family member, partner or friend, who is at risk of suicide, can be extremely frightening. It is the word that my friend used last year, when he was concerned that I had gone into a depressive low, and wondered if I might be at risk of a suicide attempt: "I'm starting to feel very frightened for you."

Supportive family and friends, who are trying to understand, have a huge role to play.

Not everyone will understand, though. When I first became suicidal in March 2012, my closest friend, at the time, reacted with a sense of shock and incomprehension: "But you're such a strong person." "You're a happy person. You're always smiling."

He saw my descent into suicidal crisis as a weakness. In addition, he was deeply religious, and saw my suicidal intent as a sin. "You have the devil inside you," he said.

Although I have no religious faith, this was still very difficult to hear. I had recently experienced the terror of believing that there may be 'dark forces' within the house, and so his comment was highly unsettling.

He continued to provide practical help, offering to give me lifts to places. I think he felt many conflicting emotions, torn between wanting to help, and feeling dismayed and disappointed in me, and struggling to accept that his friend had, in his eyes, succumbed to demonic impulses. He gradually withdrew from me and, although we are still on amicable terms, and communicate occasionally via social media, we never see each other now.

My close friends are now entirely different from those that I had in 2012.

I found that family members sometimes reacted with a sense of denial, and they strove to 'normalise' the situation and minimise the severity of what was happening. Despite the fact that I had made several suicide attempts and had been admitted to psychiatric hospital, a relative said: "Oh, you'll be all right." I think it is perhaps that the acceptance of the reality of the situation would be too painful and frightening and so, in order to protect herself, she minimised the severity of the situation and the risks.

For carers and family members who are aware of the risks to their loved one, the stress and fear can be overwhelming. On many occasions I have been contacted by a family member or partner of a client, and have witnessed the profound distress and sense of powerlessness that they experience.

I recall how the partner of one of our clients came to see me at our Suicide Crisis Centre and broke down in tears, because she was so fearful that her loved one would die. Although our remit is to support people who are at risk of suicide, we also need to respond to those who are caring for them, and recognise the emotional impact upon them. Carers and family members would much rather experience this emotional impact, and do all they can to help the person to survive, than not know that the person is at risk, but it is important that they receive support, too. The suicidal person should not feel guilt at sparking this distress in the people who care for them. Those who care would much rather experience it, and have you alive, than lose you to suicide.

Her partner had been coming in to see us every day, at our Suicide Crisis Centre, during the crisis period. They have now both emerged from that extremely dark period and say their relationship is stronger than it ever was before.

Some of the family members and friends of our clients may have no idea that the person is a suicide risk. The client has told no one, apart from us. It is concerning that a person can hide their suicidal intent so well. The client may feel that they don't want to cause stress and anxiety to their loved ones. Occasionally a client will feel that those around them won't understand or may react in an unhelpful way. And men will often cite a wish to present a "strong" façade to the world, because they feel a pressure, within society, to do this. They feel it is expected of them.

The many references to "strength" and "weakness", when discussing suicidality, can be so unhelpful. It is even the case that many social media pages dedicated to suicide prevention display the phrase: "Stay strong." The phrase makes me so uncomfortable. It seems to provide no encouragement to be open about the fact that you may be finding life incredibly difficult, and that your ability to function well is diminishing. The phrase doesn't encourage you to seek help, but rather suggests that you should be able to help yourself. By simply "staying strong", you'll get through it. I wish we could feel that it is absolutely okay to collapse under the weight of extreme pressure, traumatic events, or when life overwhelms you. We don't have to always be "strong". People should feel able to show their vulnerability because it enables them to be helped.

Indeed, it takes massive courage to seek help. I have seen how apprehensive some of our clients are, when they first come to see us and they are sitting in the reception area. One of our clients told me how he had arrived at our Crisis Centre, and had found it so difficult to come into the building. He had been pacing outside, and a member of staff went out to encourage him to come inside. He sat waiting for a few moments in reception, wondering whether he had done the right thing, and feeling a strong desire to make his escape.

There is huge bravery in making yourself vulnerable and revealing that you are in crisis.

I have noticed that many of our male clients say that they do not feel that they would be able to be supported by more than one member of our team. It is perhaps that it has been so difficult to open up to one person, that the thought of having to go through the process with another person feels too much. One of our clients expressed this very directly: "If you had told me, after our first appointment, that you were passing me on to someone else, I wouldn't have felt able to come back."

In my experience, our female clients feel more able to have two or more people involved in their care than male clients.

A client who is apprehensive about coming to our Crisis Centre might choose to email or text us initially. It allows them to build up a connection with us first, and start to feel that they can trust us. This communication may go on for a few days until they are ready to come into our Crisis Centre. For some clients, it is easier for them to express deep emotions in writing, rather than face to face. It is sometimes their email communication, in those initial few days, that gives the most detail of their situation and, crucially, the impact upon them. They may be able to write information that they would struggle to express in a face to face meeting.

Some clients continue to find it helpful to email between appointments precisely because they find it easier to write about complex and upsetting situations, than talk about them. It is also a way of keeping connected with us. One of our clients lived a long way from our centre and his work commitments made it difficult for him to come in to see us every day. So he emailed every day. He later told us that he used to imagine that the person supporting him was in front of him and he wrote as if he was talking to her.

Other clients find text support between appointments helpful. In 2012, when a clinician suggested to me that this form of support could be helpful and that I should consider texting a charity when I was feeling suicidal, I was sceptical that it would help. But it definitely can help, if the client knows the team that they are texting. A huge amount can be expressed in texts.

One of my favourite texts that I receive from clients has simply one word: "Morning." It's generally a sign that they are not currently in crisis, and just want to keep connected with us. For me, it's a beautiful reminder that they are still here, still alive.

Our male clients, in particular, seem to find email and text support helpful. Our charity has consistently had a high proportion of male clients, and it is often the case that more than 50% of our clients are male, and sometimes as high as 75 or 80%. It would be interesting to do detailed research on why so many men feel able to access our services, since there is often a belief that men may be more reluctant to seek help than women.

Our independence may be part of the reason that men come to us. I have already touched upon the fact that some men fear going to their GP because it will mean that a record remains of the reason for their visit and they believe that it may impact upon their future job prospects. There is also the issue of many of our male clients finding it difficult to be supported by more than one person. That is incredibly difficult for most crisis organisations to provide. There is also the flexibility of our service and the level of control that our clients have – they decide how often they come in to see us, and what forms of support they receive.

A significant number of male clients come to us after a relationship breakup. One man came to us after his wife told him that she was leaving him, after decades of marriage. He felt that there were no warning signs that it was going to happen. It happened very suddenly. She announced that she was leaving him, and she left that day. If he had felt, for some time, that there were difficulties in the relationship, then he would have felt less of a sense of shock, but he had seen no indications of it. She told him that she had met someone else and that she would be moving in with him.

Throughout his life, he had been the person that everyone depended upon, he told us. For the first time, he felt utterly destabilised. He knew he needed to seek help, but had no idea where to go. He ruled out his GP, because he felt that any suggestion of mental health issues might mean that he was considered unable to continue in the profession that he worked in.

He almost never watched television, he told us. By chance, he walked into a room where a television was on. It was a regional news programme, and he told me that an item about Suicide Crisis came on which explained about our Suicide Crisis Centre. In the days that followed he tried to dismiss what he had seen, but it kept coming back to him and he made contact with us. He subsequently told us that he felt that he was meant to see the television news item and find us.

It was apparent that he had been having 'absent' spells, since his wife had left, which sounded like dissociation. There were periods of time that he could recall nothing about, and friends had been telling him that there were times when it appeared that he was in a trance, and they could get no reaction from him. On one occasion, he told us that he had suddenly found himself on a road one night, with a lorry driver shouting words of abuse at him, because he had stepped out into the road and the driver had narrowly missed him. He had no recollection of how he got there. On another occasion, he found himself at the end of his road in his slippers. In one of the most frightening episodes, he awoke to find himself holding a knife in each hand. I contacted one of our clinical advisers who works within psychiatric services and she agreed that it sounded like dissociation. We were both very concerned about him because of the risks that it was posing to him.

He made a decision to barricade himself into his room at night to make it more difficult to leave the house, or collect items that might be harmful to him.

The loss of his wife was akin to experiencing a bereavement, he told me. Indeed it seemed to reawaken intensely painful feelings of loss for close relatives who had died in recent years: his father and his older brother. There was a sense that he had not been able to mourn them, or acknowledge the turbulent emotions that the circumstances of their deaths evoked. In the weeks and months after their deaths, he had been supporting everyone else, suppressing his own grief. Now it was as if "all the boxes were open." It was as if, in the past, he had locked all the painful events in boxes in his mind. He described how the ending of his marriage "blew the lids off all the other boxes." It was as if all his previous pain and loss, that he had suppressed, in order to take care of his other family members, had now been uncovered.

He was still caring for other close family members but felt utterly alone. His trust in other human beings had been shattered and he could not imagine building relationships with other people in the future.

His self-esteem and sense of worth were profoundly affected by his wife leaving him. He felt that his physical appearance may have been the root cause for her leaving. Prior to her departure, he had never felt insecure about his appearance. Now he couldn't bear to look at himself in the mirror.

I recall the day he came to see me and told me that he had trialled his suicide method.

I feared that we would lose this decent, caring, sensitive man, who had such a good heart and who had conducted himself with such dignity in the aftermath of his marriage breakup, demonstrating generosity of spirit towards his ex-wife and prioritising his family's needs over his own.

Despite the immense difficulty of trusting anyone, after what he had experienced, he was able to trust us, and remained under our care for several months, until he felt ready to leave.

Trust is a massive issue for so many of our clients. Wounded by people and by life, they fear the consequences of trusting again, and protect themselves fiercely. I see how guarded they may be, during their initial appointment with us.

One of our recent clients spoke very little at his first appointment. He referred to a recent relationship where trust had been breached, which, he said, left him unable to trust other people. He was extremely isolated, and even appeared isolated from the family members with whom he had had a close relationship until recently.

When he came in again two days later, it was clear that there had been a significant deterioration in his mood. He felt that he was likely to make a suicide attempt that evening, and so I contacted his GP surgery while he was with me, as he appeared to be showing signs of clinical depression. The on-call GP offered him an appointment half an hour later at the surgery, but my client was not prepared to go. He felt there was no point. The GP was aware of this and said the appointment would remain there, if he wanted it. The GP also commented that my client ("M") seemed to frequently reject offers of help. I thought, but did not say: "He is rejecting them because they are not the right kind of help for him. It is not that he does not want to be helped."

I arranged to phone M that evening at a fixed time, so that he and I could determine what would be our best course of action, to ensure that he stayed safe. When I called, he was feeling more settled, and did not feel that he would make an attempt that night. He had the overnight emergency number, if he felt at risk during the night or in the early hours of the morning.

The night passed quietly, but in the middle of the following afternoon, he called us and it was clear, immediately, that there was an imminent risk of a suicide attempt. He asked me if I could help him to get into hospital because he would attempt, if he remained where he was. He was ready to leave the house to carry out his plans. He told me that he would not attempt suicide in the house, because he had a dog, who he loved and treasured, and he would not want his dog to find his body.

I called 999 and was told that an ambulance would be sent out. I thought that it would be with him within minutes, but time passed and no ambulance had arrived. I spoke to M about my calling a taxi to take him to the general hospital, but he didn't want that. He felt the delay in sending out an ambulance reflected the fact that he was considered a low priority – that his life didn't matter. I called 999 again to ask what was happening and was told that they had been inundated with calls for ambulances that afternoon, and could give no time frame for an ambulance response. M was becoming increasingly agitated, and stated that he was "going for a walk". I understood this to mean a walk to the place where he would end his life, and, when I explored this with him, he confirmed that this is what he meant. I redialled 999 and requested that the police attend as he was about to leave home with the intention of killing himself. The police stayed on the phone to me, silently, while I continued to talk to M. M now felt a greater sense of urgency and was stating that he was going to the shed at the bottom of his garden, where he had the means to end his life. It would be quicker, he said. He could do it within minutes.

M quietly asked me to give up on him and to let him go. He told me that he was in unbearable emotional pain and asked me to let him be released from his suffering, and to let him die. I gently told him that I could never give up on a client and that I could never stop trying to help a client to survive. He terminated the call. I urged the police to hurry because he was going to the shed to kill himself. Minutes passed, and then the police arrived.

He was admitted to hospital, and, despite being extremely vulnerable in the days that followed, he slowly started to recover. He is starting to learn to trust again, having realised that there are people on whom he can rely, and who will not let him down.

Increasingly, we are being contacted by people from all over the country. Despite the fact that we currently only offer services in Gloucestershire, we have an internet presence, and people find us. We have taken calls from as far away as Yorkshire, Edinburgh and the Shetland Isles. Although we cannot take distant callers on as clients (as they cannot come to us and we cannot travel to them) we provide immediate help.

When people call from a distance, it is often because they are at a location where they intend to attempt suicide. We need to involve emergency services in their area, whilst remaining in contact with the person at risk.

Our most recent distance call was from a young man in London, who was on his way to the place where he intended to end his life. He was communicating with us by phone calls and texts, and, during the text communication, I was able to alert the police. While I was on the phone to them he sent me a text, asking if I had contacted the police. I mentioned this to the police call handler, and she instructed me to tell him that I hadn't called them.

I paused and said: "I'm sorry, I can't do that. I can't lie to him. I can avoid answering the question, or give an ambiguous answer, but I cannot lie to him."

I knew about the importance of honesty. I knew the impact upon me of reading my psychiatric records and knowing that I had been told untruths, on several occasions, by clinicians who had been in contact with me. If you lie to a client or patient, you may lose their trust forever. It may mean that they never use your services again. I never want our clients to experience that loss of trust that I felt, which led me to disengage totally from mental health care in our county.

The police were able to intercept him on his way to the location, ensuring his safety.

He contacted us later that day to thank us. He wasn't angry about the police involvement, and said that he knew that it was done out of care for him.

The contact that we have from people who are outside our county indicates the need for Crisis Centres all over the country. People who are in crisis know this. However, it is not those of us who have experienced crisis who usually make these decisions. The decision-makers may have a very different perspective, sadly.

It is the psychiatrists and professors who the decision-makers usually turn to, with regard to all aspects of suicide prevention. They are the ones advising and suggesting initiatives. If a psychiatrist and a professor had been the inspiration behind a Suicide Crisis Centre in Gloucestershire, I believe it would be a very different Crisis Centre from that which we have created. It would have to be. The decision-makers and people of influence in the county would have loved it, though.

A South West suicide initiative has been set up recently, which is led by a psychiatrist. I attended one of their events recently, where the keynote speaker was an eminent professor. Before he spoke, the psychiatrist emphasised the professor's importance in the field of suicide prevention and went on to explain that, if the professor had an opinion about something, then a huge proportion of people would automatically take that as their opinion, too. He explained this with the phrase: "If he thinks it, then I think it."

This was said to emphasise his eminent status in suicide prevention, but it concerned me a little. I wondered why they automatically took his view as their own, and why they didn't perhaps explore the issue themselves, which might lead them to having a different view. It concerned me that this approach might hinder opportunities for original thought, and for questioning and challenging of established opinions.

I feel that there are no 'experts', as such, and that no one has the definitive answers. There is a widely-used term "Expert by Experience", which is used to describe people with lived experience. I have never felt comfortable with this. We are all learning continually, and acquiring more knowledge. That includes professors and psychiatrists, as well as people with lived experience. I would never wish to be called an "Expert by Experience". I learn more every day from our clients and from the situations that arise. My greatest learning has come from them.

However much a professor may know, he will not know everything and, if his opinion is taken as gospel, then we lose so many possibilities for new ideas and new initiatives. We may be able to think beyond what he is saying and consider something that he may not have explored yet. All these opportunities are lost, if we simply make his opinion our opinion.

We need to be able to reconsider and challenge our own opinions and ideas, too, as we gain more knowledge or learn by experience.

On so many occasions, our clients have shown us the way that we need to develop services. Our outreach work and overnight emergency line came into existence because of their expressed need for these services. We had a model of how to run our services, but they showed us that we needed to do even more, and include additional services. This demonstrates how we may need to be prepared to divert from the ideas we had, or to incorporate additional ideas.

Virtually no one thought it possible that a recently suicidal woman could set up a Suicide Crisis Centre. If this unlikely outcome can be achieved, then so much more must be possible. There must be so many more ideas and initiatives that have yet to be uncovered, that can help to reduce the number of people who die by suicide. I wonder if they will be derided and rejected, as my ideas were, or whether they will be encouraged and nurtured. We have no idea what possibilities we may lose, if we are not prepared to think beyond the usual.

My experiences have shown me that those of us with mental health diagnoses can be underestimated and devalued. Our abilities may go unnoticed and our potential may be doubted. It means that we may have to fight extraordinarily hard to be heard, or have our ideas taken seriously. I sometimes feel that the powerful, influential people in my county were so blinded by the red flashing light of my diagnosis that they were unable to see me as a capable individual, or see the potential of my ideas.

In the early days of setting up our charity, I remember talking to the leader of another charity in the county. She told me: "You do not have to answer your critics and doubters verbally. Let your work speak for itself."

It was such excellent advice. The results of our work answer the critics and doubters in a far more powerful way than I ever could verbally.

It has been an extraordinary journey for me. I sometimes sit quietly and wonder how any of it has been possible.

From the darkness and chaos of destabilising trauma, I was propelled into a new and unrecognisable world of unimaginable emotional and physical pain, which I thought I would never be able to endure or survive. But those experiences have taken me to a place where I have found something so meaningful and important to me, in the form of our charity, that I cannot imagine doing anything else.

It is perhaps through the most extreme and painful experiences that we are able to learn, grow and develop most as people.

My colleagues and I have been alongside our clients as they travel through the dark landscape of their journey, too. Their pain is intense and, like me, they do not know at the time how they will survive it. I am so thankful that they have survived.

We know that our clients will have a positive impact upon the world. I have yet to meet a client who was not fundamentally caring and giving. I see such kind, sensitive, courageous individuals. We witness the very best of human nature. They will go out into the world and affect people in a positive way. That is a source of hope.

Our clients usually tell me that their greatest wish is that they can help other people in the future. I know that they will.

They are our hope for the future.

Our clients are the quiet but powerful voice that demonstrates that Suicide Crisis works. I hope that they are being heard. In the same way that it was obvious to me that a Suicide Crisis Centre needed to be set up here, it seems obvious to me that we need Suicide Crisis Centres in other parts of the country.

Clients tell us that they would not have survived, if it were not for our charity. That is such a powerful statement and a reason, surely, to look at opening Crisis Centres elsewhere.

I would like to leave the final word to Al, one of our clients, who expressed his feelings about our charity:-

"What you have set up works. What you are doing and how you do it works. I am still here as proof and I know that without you there is a very good chance that I would not have been."

This book is dedicated to all our clients, past, present and future.

It is also a tribute to Juliet.

My thanks to our clients who gave permission for their stories to be included anonymously, and to Juliet's family.

An exceptional team of individuals support our clients, and I am indebted to them, and to all my colleagues.

Lightning Source UK Ltd.
Milton Keynes UK
UKHW020815280220
359458UK00013B/199